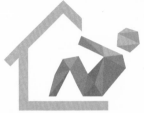

The Bodyweight Home Workout
Journal

Your pocket personal trainer for at-home workouts.

Created with love by:

Amir Atighehchi, Ariel Banayan, Mikey Ahdoot,
& The Habit Nest Team

For information about permission to reproduce elections from this book, email **team@habitnest.com**

Visit our website at **habitnest.com**

Publishers Disclaimer

While the publisher and author have used their best efforts in preparing this book, they make no representations or warranties with respect to the accuracy or completeness of the contents of this book. The advice and strategies contained herein may not be suitable for your situation. You should consult with a professional where appropriate. Neither the publisher nor the author shall be liable for any loss of profit or any other commercial damages, including but not limited to special, incidental, consequential, or other damages. The company, product, and service names used in this book are for identification purposes only. All trademarks and registered trademarks are the property of their respective owners.

Special Thanks

We'd like to extend a wholehearted, sincere thank you to the Habit Nest team for all their help in bringing this project to life. Learn more about us here: **habitnest.com/pages/about-us**

We love ya!

Exercises Disclaimer

The exercises provided by Habit Nest™ (and habitnest.com) are meant to serve as a general guide and are not to be interpreted as a recommendation for a specific treatment plan, product, or course of action. The exercises provided are not without their risks, and this or any other exercise program may result in injury. They include, but are not limited to: risk of injury, aggravation of a pre-existing condition, or adverse effect of over-exertion such as muscle strain, abnormal blood pressure, fainting, disorders of heartbeat, and very rare instances of heart attack. To reduce the risk of injury, before beginning this or any exercise program, please consult a healthcare provider for appropriate exercise prescription and safety precautions. While this is an exercise guide, it is not intended to be a direct fit for each person. It is imperative that each person tweaks the program to work for them in a way that suits their personal needs best, especially from a safety standpoint. Do not perform any exercises that cause you pain in any way. Consult with a certified personal trainer to help guide you through each exercise in person to assure they are all being done properly and in ways that will minimize injury.

This content is provided as is and in no way intended as a substitute for medical consultation. Habit Nest™ disclaims any liability from and in connection with this program. As with any exercise program, if at any point during your workout you begin to feel faint, dizzy, or have physical discomfort, you should stop immediately and consult a physician.

Information Disclaimer

The information provided by Habit Nest™ (and habitnest.com) is for educational and entertainment purposes only, and is not to be interpreted as a recommendation for a specific treatment plan, product, or course of action. Habit Nest™ does not provide specific medical advice, and is not engaged in providing medical services. Habit Nest™ does not replace consultation with a qualified health or medical professional who sees you in person, for the health and medical needs of yourself or a loved one. In addition, while Habit Nest™ frequently updates its contents, medical, health and fitness information changes rapidly, and therefore, some information may be out of date. Please see a physician or health professional immediately if you suspect you may be ill or injured. Before implementing any nutritional information provided, consult with a nutritionist as well to make sure you can fit your personal health and nutrition needs.

ISBN: 9781950045235

Second Edition

The Habit Nest Mission

We are a team of people obsessed with taking ACTION
and learning new things as quickly as possible.

We love finding the fastest, most effective ways to build
a new skill, then systemizing that process for others.

With building new habits, we empathize with others every step of the way
because we go through the same process ourselves. We live and breathe
everything in our company.

We use our hard-earned intuition to outline beautifully designed, intuitive
products to help people live happier, more fulfilled lives.

Everything we create comes with a mix of bite-sized information, strategy,
and accountability. This hands you a simple yet drastically effective roadmap
to build any skill or habit with.

We take this a step further by diving into published
scientific studies, the opinions of subject-matter experts, and the feedback we
get from customers to further enhance all the products we create.

Ultimately, Habit Nest is a practical, action-oriented startup aimed at helping
others take back decisional authority over every action they take.

We're here to help people live wholesome, rewarding lives at the brink of their
potential!

– Amir Atighehchi, Ari Banayan, & Mikey Ahdoot.
Cofounders of Habit Nest

Contents

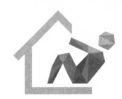

Our Mission in Creating This Journal

Sometimes, it isn't easy to motivate yourself to exercise.

Sometimes when you decide to work out, you don't feel like pushing yourself.

Sometimes, you need a gym buddy at home.

Our goal in creating this journal was to make it as easy as possible for you to get moving, have an amazing workout, watch incredibly fast progress happen right before your eyes, and ultimately feel supremely confident in your body.

We created this all-in-one personal trainer & tracker so that you don't have do ANY thinking when it comes to your workouts.

Having this journal removes any possible excuse for experiencing an awesome workout, because the journal itself provides a way for you to be competitive with yourself so you can continue to see progress, without plateauing.

There is no guess-work. Your ONLY mission is to actually get your workout clothes on and open the book. If you can make the commitment to get into exercise mode, open the book, and start the first exercise, you'll find yourself pushing harder than ever before without even realizing how it happened.

We created this journal to help you actually achieve your ultimate fitness goals.

The Key Factors
of Training Success

How the Journal Works

Every day, you're going to be given a COMPLETE workout routine designating:

- **Which muscles** will be worked,

- **Exactly which workouts to do** (each will come with complete explanations, guiding images, and alternative exercises),

- **How many sets you'll do** (how many times you'll begin and end a complete round of an exercise) of each workout, and

- **The rep range** (the number of contractions) **you're aiming for** on each set.

What to Do Each Day

You have two tasks to complete every day you choose to workout:

1. Before you start working out :

Look at what the day's workout consists of, i.e., which exercises you'll be completing. Then, read the explanations and images in the workout index in the back of the journal for those exercises.

To make it even easier, we included exercise guide links in the top left corner of each workout. These include the workout descriptions for that day.

Until you're familiar with each exercise, it'll be annoying to keep looking back to the index during your workout.

It would be wise to get familiar with the exercises the night before or for a couple minutes before you begin.

2. During your workout:

For each exercise, fill in the number of reps you complete. This is the most adequate way to track your progress.

We designate tracking lines for all of this, you just have to write down the numbers.

We'll be aiming to complete 3 sets per exercise. There are a series of ways to challenge yourself as you progress through the journal as well.

You can up the sets completed from 3 to 4 per exercise (we included tracking for this on each workout page).

Push & Pull Muscle Groups

The combination of muscles that will be worked on any given day will vary. In general, we'll combine one 'push' muscle with one 'pull' muscle rather than the traditional method of using multiple 'pull' or 'push' muscles.

The 'push' muscles are those which require a pushing action from the body to complete a movement. The most simple example is a push up. The 'pull' muscles are those that require a pulling motion – the back and biceps are examples of pull muscles.

The reason we'll regularly combine one 'push' and one 'pull' muscle in each day's workout is that we'll be getting more of the body involved on a regular basis.

Tracking Your Progress

Bodyweight training is about using our own bodies to contract our muscles under tension to stimulate growth, strength, power, and endurance.

The factors that determine the quality of our body's reaction to the training we put it through are:

1. Frequency
(How often we train)

2. Intensity
(How hard we train)

3. Time
(How long we train)

4. Type of exercise
(What we do when we train)

All of this boils down to one very simple principle:

Our bodies change when we regularly push our current limits. The moment your level of intensity becomes 'normal' is the moment you stop changing.

If you're currently working out one day per week, then increasing to 2 or 3 times a week will have a significant impact on your progress.

If you already work out 4–5 times a week, you have to find alternate ways to increase intensity and push the limit to continue changing at the rate you want.

Between the four factors above, you always have something available to use that can increase the intensity with which you face your body's progress.

If you can continuously reach the point where you're really pushing the boundary of what your body is capable of, you'll always be making strides towards your goals.

This journal will help you consistently find that boundary - it's up to you to push past it.

Resting Periods Between Sets

It is important to pay attention to how much rest you take in between sets.

You need to give your muscles enough time to be ready for the next set while making sure you're not wasting time and are working with *maximum intensity*.

You'll need to find the proper balance for yourself. Your resting periods will decrease the more experienced you become.

In general, 30 seconds – 90 seconds in between sets is a good benchmark.

Anything under may be too short, and anything over is probably too long.

What's important is that you learn to recognize when you're wasting time out of laziness and to limit that as much as possible!

How Often Should I Exercise?

This is a common question that is situational based on what's realistic for each person.

The journal is undated and structured to be used by what works for you, your goals, and your schedule.

As a frame of reference:

Light:
Exercise 2 days a week.

Medium:
Exercise 4 days a week.

Hard:
Exercise 5-6 days a week.

If you're driven enough to achieve the best results, you should set a long-term goal of building up to 5-6 workouts a week.

Targeting Each Part of Every Muscle

The muscles we focus on in bodyweight training are the **Chest, Back, Shoulders, Biceps, Triceps, Trapezius, Quadriceps, Hamstrings, Glutes, Calves, and Abdominal Muscles.**

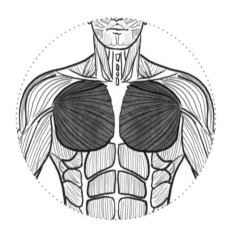

Chest

The chest (pectoral muscle) is one of the bigger muscles on the upper part of our body. As such, no one workout will adequately target the entire chest area.

Chest workouts will either *mainly* target the upper chest, middle part of the chest, or the lower chest. Focusing on all three major areas will allow the muscle to develop fully for maximum growth, thickness, and strength.

Back

The back covers an enormous part of our upper body and, like the chest, will require many different types of exercises to ensure that each part is being targeted adequately.

Back workouts are generally split into those that target the latissimus dorsi ('lats' or 'wings;' the muscles behind your abdomen) and exercises that target the muscles closer to the top of our backs(the entire area in between our shoulder blades).

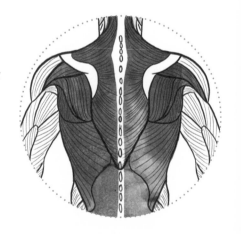

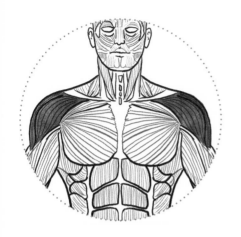

Shoulders

Shoulder development is crucially important in bodyweight training, partially because shoulder development improves the way the biceps, triceps, chest, and back look.

More importantly, the shoulders are at work when performing most upper-body exercises and thus need to be strong enough to perform those exercises without risking injury.

Shoulder workouts generally work the entire muscle. However, the muscle is split into three distinct parts - front, medial, and lateral, which all require unique workouts to develop the muscle in its totality.

Biceps

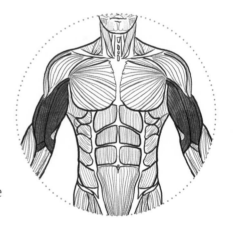

As one of the smaller muscles on our bodies, the biceps tire out more quickly than bigger muscles like the chest or back, and, due to muscle size, simply cannot grow as strong.

Bicep workouts will focus on making sure we hit the long-head and short-head of the muscle (inner and outer parts).

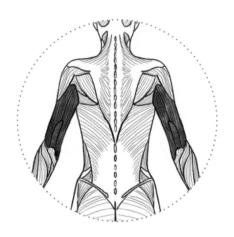

Triceps

Tricep development is really important to arm strength and size because the tricep makes up more than 50% (around 2/3rds) of your arm. Triceps have 3 'heads' (hence the name) - lateral, medial and long. Most workouts hit all 3, but each requires unique attention, which we'll definitely give them!

Abs, Obliques & Core

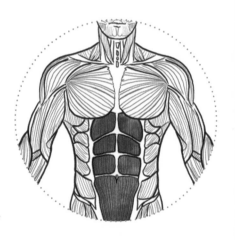

Your abdominal muscles consist of the rectus abdominis (six-pack), external obliques, and internal obliques. Abs are smaller muscles and require less training, but as smaller muscles, the recovery periods are also shorter - meaning you can train them more often.

The most important aspect in having visible abs is your body fat percentage, which is largely a result of the quality of your diet.

So we WILL train abs, but whether they show or not will be very dependent on how clean you eat.

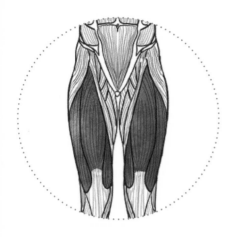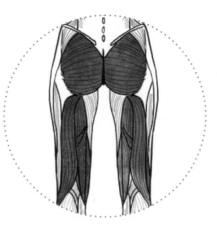

Legs

Our leg muscles are split into three general parts - quadriceps, hamstrings (and glutes), and calves.

We'll do bigger compound workouts that work the entire leg, but also do exercises to focus on each part of the leg individually.

Leg training is critically important because it boosts testosterone, allowing further growth of the rest of the body. Don't think when you're doing legs you're missing out on doing something that shows more.

Our lower bodies are a big part of how we look. They give the body the foundation it needs for healthy and active living and in fact allow the muscles on the upper body to grow.

Mind-Muscle Connection

"What puts you over the top? It is the mind that actually creates the body, it is the mind that really makes you work out... it is the mind that visualizes what the body ought to look like as the finished product."

– Arnold Schwarzenegger

The idea behind the mind-muscle connection is simple:

The more your mind is focused on the muscle being worked as it contracts, the greater your muscle development will be.

Acetylcholine is a neurotransmitter that stimulates your muscles to move.

The more you bring an active attention to the muscle being worked, the contraction in each and every rep, the more acetylcholine that's produced. The more acetylcholine that's produced, the better the contraction, and the better the gains.

Therefore... **focused attention is very, very important.**

You can't study when your mind is wandering, right? You can't be productive when your thoughts aren't with what you're doing. Working out your body is no different - active attention on what you're doing is essential.

Bring the importance of the mind-muscle connection to your attention at the very beginning of every workout and try to remember it throughout each set.

Become a Strategic Stretcher

Stretching is commonly done improperly (e.g. stretching muscles that are already overstretched) **or is often ignored altogether**.

Instead of stretching random muscles, we recommend becoming a strategic stretcher. This means figuring out which of your muscles are tightest and have mobility issues, then stretching those specifically.

For example, if you have anterior pelvic tilt (a common issue, look it up if you're unfamiliar!), you would want to **stretch the following muscles:**

· Hip flexors
· Thoracic spine
· Lower back

And **avoid stretching:**
· Hamstrings

You'll also want to strengthen specific muscles that are weak and underused, leading to poor posture / mobility. In the example above, you'd want to strengthen your upper back (specifically the erector spinaei), your abs, and your glutes.

A fantastic resource for mobility exercises (and fitness in general) is the *Athlean-X* channel on YouTube. Jeff Cavaliere, the founder, has created many in-depth and science-based videos on improving mobility for specific body parts.

The Extreme Importance of Form

Before beginning any exercise, you have to be absolutely sure that you adequately understand how to complete the exercise without getting injured.

We provide explanations of each exercise in the back of this journal, but if you're ever unclear, it only takes 30 seconds to look any exercise up online!

Our bodies are masters of compensation.
Where the body can cheat, it will.

There must be a conscious vigilance to retain proper form.
And let's be very clear: Form is **vitally** important.

Without Proper Form:

1. There is always a *risk of injury*.

2. You're most likely *missing the target muscle* because you're *compensating with body parts that don't need to be used*.

There is zero reason not to use proper form on any given exercise.

We will explain what proper form is for every exercise we provide in the journal, **but if you're ever unclear, PLEASE search online for a video that delves further into how to perform the workout properly until you're confident you can complete it without getting hurt.**

Check your ego at the door, and make sure you can complete every rep of each exercise with **the right form.**

Not completing a rep because you're exhausted and can't do it without breaking form is one thing – a beautiful thing.

Hurting yourself to complete a rep with muscles that aren't supposed to be involved is another thing – an ugly thing.

Do the beautiful thing.

Bonus Tip:
A commonly ignored yet incredibly useful strategy is to record yourself doing a specific exercise so you can actually SEE your form vs. tracking it mentally.

What's the Deal with Cardio?

Look, cardiovascular and aerobic exercise are always important – both for overall health as well as weight loss/muscle development.

Traditional aerobic exercise (static exercise like running on a treadmill, biking, or using the elliptical machine) is obviously great for health purposes, but it is not the optimal cardiovascular work for burning fat.

HIIT Cardio:

To really derive the benefit of keeping healthy on the inside while burning the most fat, we recommend HIIT cardio 2-3 times a week.

It's all about short bursts of intensity rather than longer, static routines.

One day per week of this journal is dedicated to doing a cardio routine which is likely different from your ordinary idea of what cardio should be.

We'll give you a specific routine of circuit exercises that you'll perform (in order) with very short rest periods (or none at all).

It helps keep you engaged, works on muscle toning while getting your heart rate up, and makes cardio just a little bit easier to do with a smile on your face.

If you're vehemently opposed to doing cardio, an approach you can take is an experimental one – try doing minimal cardio for 2-3 weeks (just the days in the journal, nothing extra) and see what happens to your body fat % over time. If your nutrition + body-sculpting intensity is spot-on, and you're not burning as much fat as you'd like, you can introduce additional cardio days then.

Alternatively, if you want to guarantee your results and get maximum effectiveness off the bat and not risk wasting any time, start with the above suggestion of 2-3 cardio days a week for 20 minutes a session. Add an additional day per week if you're not seeing great fat loss results.

Cardio is a key factor to deploy when your fat loss is stalling – use it strategically, wisely, and without complaints.

The Importance of Workout Intensity

The truth is, you need to have a very high level of intensity when body-sculpting to see real progress. **Remember, intensity is what makes or breaks a workout, every day.**

However, this is a VERY easy point to misread and not understand properly. The level of intensity you should push yourself to build in your workouts looks like:

- Establishing the mentality of giving your ALL to the workout, not wasting a second or moment and moving with a fiery, powerful sense of direction.

- Having complete mental focus to perform your absolute best each day.

- Minimizing distractions like using your phone during rest periods.

- Tracking your rest periods and not letting them linger on past 45-120 seconds. This may mean starting a set when you feel too tired to do it at your best, but doing it anyways.

- Having pure mental focus on maintaining proper form and pushing your body to its limit with each set (without risking injury to yourself).

- Pushing yourself to set NEW limits by challenging yourself to do an extra rep when you feel completely dead after a set (again, while prioritizing staying safe and avoiding injury).

- Removing the fear of not hitting your desired rep range and feeling like a failure; knowing that your true goal is to give each set everything you've got and reach muscle failure.

- Not showing your body mercy if it feels tired / craves long rest periods. Force yourself to push through and you will feel more energized.

If you feel it's naturally difficult to achieve all this, know that reaching the proper intensity in your workouts is absolutely a *trainable habit* within yourself. Make it a long-term goal to challenge yourself to reach it.

To help hold you accountable to increasing your intensity, we added a 'Workout Intensity' tracker at the end of each workout where you can record how intense your effort was each day as a numerical rating out of 10.

Adequate Recovery

Soreness is **GOOD!**

You **WILL** feel sore.

You **WANT** to feel sore – that's one way you know you're doing work. As you progress through this journal, you will notice your stamina and workout capacity increasing.

But that being said, recovery is a necessity. Pushing yourself to the limit is also necessary.

How do I find the balance?

Recovery involves more than just letting your muscles rest – it involves letting your joints, connective tissues, and bones rest as well. There is lots more involved in any bodyweight training exercise than just the muscle itself.

Think of it as the same reason we need to sleep every single day. Letting the body rest is enormously important.

The beautiful thing is that your body will tell you when it needs to rest! Physical exhaustion as opposed to mental fatigue becomes very obvious when the body has surpassed a certain point that you'll recognize.

Of course, that means you have to really feel the exhaustion rather than use recovery as an excuse to not push yourself or even get started with your workout.

A big part of what you gain by bodyweight training regularly is becoming sincere with yourself about when you're making excuses vs. when you really need a rest.

Regardless of how many days a week you decide to work out (we recommend 4-6 to really push yourself), getting adequate sleep is crucial to allow for proper muscle gain. If you notice your muscle growth is lower than usual, take a look at your sleep and see if you are getting enough each night based on what your body requires. Oftentimes, 8+ hours a night is optimal for enough recovery and muscle growth.

Optimizing Every Aspect of Your Nutrition

A Short Note on the Importance of Eating

You Can't Lie to Your Body.

Our bodies are machines. Machines have a few main characteristics:

1. They respond in a unique way to external stimuli.
2. They need fuel to function properly and efficiently.
3. Maintenance is required to prevent degeneration.
4. They have many component parts, each with a definite function or 'job.'
5. All the parts of a machine taken as a whole make up a unit that has one particular function in which every part plays a role.
6. They are predictable. They can be manipulated to achieve desired results.

Think about your car. You buy a car because you have a need for a method of transportation – a way to get around. The car serves this overall purpose of taking you from place to place.

But a car isn't merely a mobility device. It has many parts which each play a role in creating the possibility of being your modern day horse. In the ignition system alone there are spark plugs, ignition wire, coil and distributor that control the timing and flow of electricity to the engine's cylinders...

Every week or so, you need to get gas for the car, right? Every few months or year, your car needs to be serviced. If you want your car to be louder or faster, what do you do? You get someone to alter the exhaust system, or you change parts to increase all around power and torque.

You have a result you want to achieve... *Simply alter the machine to fit your vision.*

But you can't lie to your car. You can't tell it that you're giving it oil and give it orange juice instead.

The beauty of the human body is that it is a wonderfully intricate machine that responds mechanically to the appearance of new external stimuli, and it can be manipulated to achieve desired results the same exact way you can change the way a computer or car operates.

You can force your body to burn excess fat it holds by monitoring your macronutrient intake and obtaining the proper balance of nutrients.

But you can't tell your body to respond differently than what you put in it. Remember every day, every meal, every moment:

You cannot lie to your body.

What About Supplements?

The most important thing to realize about supplements is that they're supposed to *supplement*.

They are not necessary, and come secondary (nowhere near) the importance of training regularly with intensity and eating clean.

Supplements on their own will not change your body/do the work for you.

They can, however, help you meet your macronutrient goals, assist in muscle recovery, and help facilitate overall health, which leads to better workouts.

There is a lot of information on different types of supplements to assist in achieving your body-sculpting goals.

The two we'd like to recommend are **some form of protein powder** and **a multi-vitamin.**

If you're trying to gain muscle mass, eating enough protein is really important, and because it can be difficult to eat as much as needed, protein powder lessens the load.

Multi-vitamins simply help ensure that you're getting the basic nutrients you need even if you're not eating them!

Caloric Deficit & Macronutrient Ratios

The following is assuming that your body composition goals are to:

1. Have minimal excess body fat, and
2. Maintain or increase your body's muscle

Depending on the body you want, a proper balance needs to be struck between minimizing body fat and maintaining or increasing muscle. The food we eat is the single most important factor in both decreasing body fat and improving muscle definition.

Fat Loss vs. Weight Loss

Most people don't even scratch the surface when it comes to understanding what it means to 'lose weight.' Weight loss can come in a few different ways.

The loss of weight that shows up on a scale can either be the result of fat loss, muscle loss, or water loss.

We all have this goal of getting to an ideal weight we think will make us happy with our physique. But the number on the scale should be the least of your worries. The goal is always to be as fit as possible, be as healthy as possible, and most importantly, to be genuinely happy with your body just as it is.
The goal is to selectively manipulate the body to burn as much fat as possible, while retaining all the muscle we have on our bodies.

An example of the distinction between fat loss and weight loss is the very well-known 'no-carb' diet - complete elimination of all carbs from one's diet.

If you've heard people saying they're on a 'low-carb' or 'no-carb' diet that is working extremely well for them and quickly, here's why:

Every stored carbohydrate in your body holds 2.7 grams of water. Eliminating or seriously depriving your body of carbohydrates means you're losing a lot of water weight, which is good if you're looking to just drop the number on the scale quickly, but doesn't make sense if you want to achieve long-term weight loss and prevent future weight-gain.

There will always be people who make it work with any diet, but drastically lowering carbs for years on end isn't realistic for most people.

Achieving a Caloric Deficit

Note: Before following any nutrition advice in this journal, we recommend reaching out to your doctor and/or nutritionist to get their thoughts. This is because different people have different needs and it's always a good idea to check yours.

It's simple.

Your body needs a certain amount of energy to function.

A calorie is a unit of energy – it is the energy value of food.

When your body uses more calories than it takes in, it is forced to turn to other places to supply and fulfill the energy requirements it isn't getting from the food you're eating.
But the body has a few options for where it can go to take the energy that it needs. It can either go to fat stores, muscle protein, or a combination of both.

Our goal in achieving fat loss is to cause the body to undergo this process of finding alternate energy supplies, while doing all that we can to force the use of fat as the primary energy source rather than muscle.

When there is a caloric deficit and the body is forced to turn to alternate sources of energy, it is imperative to ensure that muscle catabolism doesn't occur.

Muscle catabolism is the breakdown of muscle tissue to supply energy for the body that isn't coming from the food we're eating. This is one of the main reasons people aren't necessarily happy with their bodies when they completely cut their carbohydrate intake.

To put everything into perspective, the moment you have a caloric surplus (you eat more calories than you burn), extra calories are stored as fat for future energy use in the event that it becomes necessary.

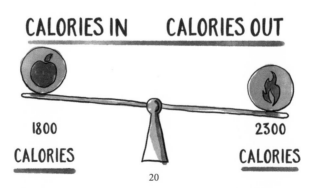

CALORIES IN   CALORIES OUT

1800 CALORIES   2300 CALORIES

Macronutrient Ratios

To lose weight, you need to eat less calories than you burn.

But the name of the game when it comes to achieving FAT loss
and preventing fat gain, is **understanding how the macronutrients you eat
affect the body.**

Regardless of the extent of your caloric deficit, if your body isn't getting what
it needs to function the way it was designed to operate, you will not be satisfied
with the way you look. Instead, you will re-gain all the weight you lose the
moment you start to eat like a human being.

The term **macronutrient** refers to the main types of food – carbohydrates,
lipids (fats), and proteins.

The **macronutrient ratio** concerns the percentage of your caloric intake each
of these three types of foods comprises.

To attain the right balance that will force your body to use fat for energy while
retaining muscle, the macronutrient intake has to be carefully plotted and it
must be tailored to your specific body type, the speed of your metabolism, and
your ordinary activity levels.

Summary

1. Your body needs energy to function, and is in a constant state of energy
   expenditure.

2. A calorie is a unit of stored energy; a measure of the value of food.

3. You can force your body to burn fat by achieving a caloric deficit.

4. A caloric deficit results where you burn more calories than you consume.

5. A caloric deficit may result in your body using muscle tissue for energy,
   which we can prevent with a proper balance of macronutrients.

Taking Action on Your Nutrition Goals

At this point, most people will take a mental note on these dietary / food points to apply going forward. But in order to **guarantee our results**, we must **guarantee we'll take action on this every day**.

As powerful as mindsets are, they are also very malleable and easily influenced by outside stimuli (like having a very common 'off day'). Meanwhile, systems (which provide accountability and tracking) are black and white - yes or no - 1 or 0.

We highly recommend putting together a structure you think can work in helping you stay consistent with your eating goals. Nothing is more demoralizing than aiming to feel better about yourself, working out hard for it, and seeing poor results (that you later justify).

After getting some clarity on which eating plan you want to follow (e.g. counting calories/macros or choosing a specific diet), there are a few ways to put it into effect.

As a free option:
You can use a dietary tracking app, Google sheet, or notepad to track calories/macros/meals. Alternatively, you can use an extra whiteboard or calendar to track whether or not you hit your goals every day. If you think you can genuinely stay consistent with this for months / the long term, this is a great option.

As a paid option:
We wrote *The Nutrition Sidekick Journal* for this exact reason - to provide a clear, unbreakable system to track your results and help you learn how to improve (without judgement!) at the same time. If a pure tracking sheet is a bit too dull, redundant, and isn't stimulating enough for you, this may be the right choice.

Some things covered inside the *Nutrition Sidekick Journal:*

1. How to manipulate your body to **burn fat while maintaining muscle.**

2. **Tracking** for your calories, water intake, and **planned meals vs. actual eaten meals.**

3. **New golden nuggets of information**, pro-tips, daily challenges, and more each day.

You can check it out at **habitnest.com/nutrition** and use discount code **TeamLean15** for **15% off** if you decide to order one.

Effectively Tracking Your Nutrition Progress

Tracking your progress is extremely important. That being said, the accuracy of your tracking is **even more important.** With flawed data that isn't actionable, your tracking is just an arbitrary, confusing, and often misleading number.

This section assumes you have two body-composition goals, which tend to be the most popular amongst people (and can be the healthiest):

1. You want to increase your muscle mass
2. You want to reach & maintain a lean body fat percentage at 8-15% (males) or 13-20% (females)

The Problem With the Scale

With bodyweight training and fat loss, the scale's results (without deeper insight on it) can be your biggest enemy. This is because our shifts in body weight are affected by SO many factors, it's impossible to identify what has changed week by week with only a weight amount.

This is where **body fat tracking** comes in, right alongside **body weight tracking**. By combining the tracking of BOTH your body fat AND the scale, you're able to see exactly HOW your weight changed from week to week - whether you gained muscle, gained body fat, lost muscle, or lost body fat.

Accurately Measuring Your Body Fat Percentage

There are many ways to do this, but the most cost-effective and practical way is to use a self-testing skinfold caliper. The one we recommend is the Accu-Measure as it costs roughly $10 on Amazon and has an existing scientific study backing up its effectiveness (it's within 1.1% accuracy of using an underwater body fat measurement, which is one of the highest levels of accuracy we have for measuring body fat).

Disclaimer: We have no affiliation with the Accu-Measure and aren't getting paid in any way for this recommendation. It's simply a great tool.

With the upsides being ease of use and cost, the biggest downsides of this method are the **potential inaccuracy** if you don't know how to measure yourself properly each week. Although it's **very possible to be incredibly accurate** with this method... it takes a good deal of practice. Thankfully, the product comes with step-by-step guide that lays out how to use it as accurately as possible.

As long as you are measuring yourself in the same location weekly, even if your placement isn't perfect, you'll be able to have comparable results you trust week after week. Make your main goal in measuring be *consistency in measuring.*

How Do I Get the Right Data?

We recommend measuring yourself weekly for both body weight (with a scale) and body fat (with the Accu-Measure).

We want to eliminate as many factors that can cause data inconsistencies as possible.

When taking your measurements, do it:

- At the same time of day (ideally mornings)
- With the same food/water intake that day (ideally none, do it right as you wake up)
- With the same amount of clothes on, and
- Without holding any objects that could throw your readings off (e.g. your phone)

You can write this data down as you progress through the journal (in the next section) or record it on a note on your phone. If you choose the latter, make sure you don't hold your phone as you're measuring yourself.

Common Misunderstandings With the Accu-Measure

After using the Accu-Measure ourselves, a few things were a bit unclear from the instruction sheet they provided. We spoke with a rep on the phone who helped clarify these points for us:

1. *Where is the iliac crest?*
To find your iliac crest, it should be near your waist line (like where you wear a belt) and you feel a big bone protruding out, towards the side of your body.

2. *How can you measure consistently and accurately?*
If you place the caliper directly on your skin, the ends will measure 2.5 inches exactly. You can use this to consistently grab the same distance each measurement.

Once you have grabbed your skin fold with your thumb and index finger, position the caliper halfway between the back of your skinfold (point closest to your body) and the front of the skinfold (point furthest from your body), 1cm away from your fingers.

Getting Even More Clarity & Reducing Measuring Inaccuracy

The most important thing with using the Accu-Measure is **measuring yourself the same way week-to-week**. Even if you're measuring yourself improperly, or the Accu-Measure itself is inaccurate, your **week-to-week changes should remain consistent** as the method of measuring is consistent.

If you want to take this to the next level, or see how close to accurate your Accu-Measure is, you can get a detailed body scan (e.g. a water displacement scan) and see how it compares to the Accu-Measure. If a discrepancy exists, you'll at least know by how much and be able to mentally keep that in mind.

Write down the following each week:

1. Measure your **total body weight** using a scale

2. Measure your **body fat %** using an Accu-Measure

3. Take your total body weight (#1) in pounds and multiply it by your body fat % (#2). This will give you your **body fat weight**.

4. Take your **total body weight** (#1) and subtract your **body fat weight** (#3) to get your **lean body mass**.

Your lean body mass consists of every part of your body that's not considered fat (muscles, tissues, bones, organs, water weight, etc.) Since a significant changing factor in weight of your lean body mass is your muscle mass, we can use lean body mass as a near-accurate measure of fluctuations in muscle gain / loss.

The biggest inconsistency with your lean body mass will be the fluctuations in your water weight. Be mindful of this and how certain factors (e.g. being dehydrated, drinking lots of water, intaking too much sodium the day before) can affect this. If something seems wrong, give it at least 2 weeks before jumping to conclusions of whether your plan is or is not working.

What Should I Do With This Measurement Data?

The next two pages provide a space to record this data weekly over a 12-week period, followed by actions steps for how to adjust weekly for each scenario. Having this data recorded next to each other will allow you to spot trends in your weekly fluctuations and make the correct adjustments of action steps based on this.

Adjusting Based On Progress

As recommended in Tom Venuto's *Burn the Fat, Feed the Muscle*, you should make the following tweaks based on your weekly fluctuations of body fat weight (B.F. Weight) and lean body mass (L.B.M.) to achieve body fat loss & muscle gain:

1. If...   B.F. Weight (↑)   L.B.M (↑)

Then: Decrease your caloric intake (recommended: 100-200) and increase your cardio.

2. If...   B.F. Weight (↓)   L.B.M (↑)

Then: This is the holy grail and we are all jealous of you. Keep doing what you're doing. This is decently rare to occur, so treat it as a huge gift if you're experiencing it!

3. If...   B.F. Weight (↑)   L.B.M (↓)

Then: This is unlikely and usually due to a measurement inaccuracy. Alternatively, this may be due to factors outside of your training and nutrition, such as being under a lot of stress and not getting adequate rest. Recheck your results, and if they're accurate, take care of yourself and see if you notice a significant difference the following week.

4. If...   B.F. Weight (↓)   L.B.M (↓)

Then: Eat more calories (recommended: 100-200) and increase protein intake if you're under 1g * your total body weight. Increasing your weight training intensity will help here as well.

This ⊖ icon means B.F. Weight L.B.M. stayed the same.

5. If...   B.F. Weight (↑)   L.B.M (⊖)

Then: Eat less calories (recommended: 100-200) and slightly increase your cardio.
Note: This action step also applies if both your L.B.M. and your body fat weight stay the same (no change as the week before).

6. If...   B.F. Weight (↓)   L.B.M

Then: This is fantastic! You're right on track, keep doing what you're doing.

Weekly Progress Tracker

Week One
Date _____

Weight .... | Body fat % ....
Fat weight .... | Lean mass ....

Adjustments

	(Circle one)	(Fill in amount)
Calories	↑ ↓ —	....
Cardio	↑ ↓ —	....
Training intensity	↑ ↓ —	....

Week Two
Date _____

Weight .... | Body fat % ....
Fat weight .... | Lean mass ....

Adjustments

	(Circle one)	(Fill in amount)
Calories	↑ ↓ —	....
Cardio	↑ ↓ —	....
Training intensity	↑ ↓ —	....

Week Three
Date _____

Weight .... | Body fat % ....
Fat weight .... | Lean mass ....

Adjustments

	(Circle one)	(Fill in amount)
Calories	↑ ↓ —	....
Cardio	↑ ↓ —	....
Training intensity	↑ ↓ —	....

Week Four
Date _____

Weight .... | Body fat % ....
Fat weight .... | Lean mass ....

Adjustments

	(Circle one)	(Fill in amount)
Calories	↑ ↓ —	....
Cardio	↑ ↓ —	....
Training intensity	↑ ↓ —	....

Week Five
Date _____

Weight .... | Body fat % ....
Fat weight .... | Lean mass ....

Adjustments

	(Circle one)	(Fill in amount)
Calories	↑ ↓ —	....
Cardio	↑ ↓ —	....
Training intensity	↑ ↓ —	....

Week Six
Date _____

Weight .... | Body fat % ....
Fat weight .... | Lean mass ....

Adjustments

	(Circle one)	(Fill in amount)
Calories	↑ ↓ —	....
Cardio	↑ ↓ —	....
Training intensity	↑ ↓ —	....

Week Seven
Date _____

Weight .... | Body fat % ....
Fat weight .... | Lean mass ....

Adjustments
	(Circle one)	(Fill in amount)
Calories	↑ ↓ —	....
Cardio	↑ ↓ —	....
Training intensity	↑ ↓ —	....

Week Eight
Date _____

Weight .... | Body fat % ....
Fat weight .... | Lean mass ....

Adjustments
	(Circle one)	(Fill in amount)
Calories	↑ ↓ —	....
Cardio	↑ ↓ —	....
Training intensity	↑ ↓ —	....

Week Nine
Date _____

Weight .... | Body fat % ....
Fat weight .... | Lean mass ....

Adjustments
	(Circle one)	(Fill in amount)
Calories	↑ ↓ —	....
Cardio	↑ ↓ —	....
Training intensity	↑ ↓ —	....

Week Ten
Date _____

Weight .... | Body fat % ....
Fat weight .... | Lean mass ....

Adjustments
	(Circle one)	(Fill in amount)
Calories	↑ ↓ —	....
Cardio	↑ ↓ —	....
Training intensity	↑ ↓ —	....

Week Eleven
Date _____

Weight .... | Body fat % ....
Fat weight .... | Lean mass ....

Adjustments
	(Circle one)	(Fill in amount)
Calories	↑ ↓ —	....
Cardio	↑ ↓ —	....
Training intensity	↑ ↓ —	....

Week Twelve
Date _____

Weight .... | Body fat % ....
Fat weight .... | Lean mass ....

Adjustments
	(Circle one)	(Fill in amount)
Calories	↑ ↓ —	....
Cardio	↑ ↓ —	....
Training intensity	↑ ↓ —	....

Getting Started

Biceps & Triceps

1. Doorway Curl

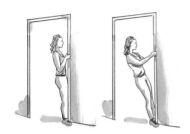

Set 1 Reps: ....14........... (Goal: 10-20)

Set 2 Reps: ....10........... (Goal: 10-20)

Set 3 Reps: ....7........... (Goal: 10-20)

Set 4 Reps: ....6........... (Goal: 10-20)
(Optional)

2. Towel Curl

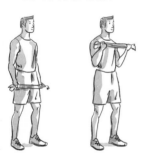

By having your 'Previous Best' reps listed for each specific exercise, you'll have a clear target to beat weekly.

Set 1 Reps: ....15........... (Goal: 10-20)

Set 2 Reps: ....12........... (Goal: 10-20)

Set 3 Reps: ....8........... (Goal: 10-20)

Set 4 Reps: ....—........... (Goal: 10-20)
(Optional)

3. Flexing Hammer Curl

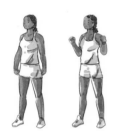

Set 1 Reps: ....13........... (Goal: 10-20)

Set 2 Reps: ....11........... (Goal: 10-20)

Set 3 Reps: ....7........... (Goal: 10-20)

Set 4 Reps: ....6........... (Goal: 10-20)
(Optional)

4. Curl Your Leg

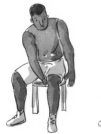 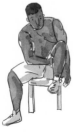

Ideally, every set should be done to failure. The suggested ranges are meant to give you a goal to aim for, but you can do more!

Set 1 Reps: ....14........... (Goal: 10-20 Each Side)

Set 2 Reps: ....12........... (Goal: 10-20 Each Side)

Set 3 Reps: ....8........... (Goal: 10-20 Each Side)

Set 4 Reps: ....6........... (Goal: 10-20 Each Side)
(Optional)

Cardio Done Today:

20 min

Biceps **& Triceps**

08 / 27 / 20
Date

1. Bodyweight Dips

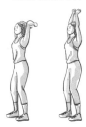

Set 1	Reps: ......12......	(Goal: 10-20)
Set 2	Reps: ......11......	(Goal: 10-20)
Set 3	Reps: ......8......	(Goal: 10-20)
Set 4 (Optional)	Reps: ......6......	(Goal: 10-20)

The fourth set on each exercise is optional but highly recommended.

2. Flexing Overhead Tricep Extension

Set 1	Reps: ......14......	(Goal: 10-20)
Set 2	Reps: ......10......	(Goal: 10-20)
Set 3	Reps: ......7......	(Goal: 10-20)
Set 4 (Optional)	Reps: ......—......	(Goal: 10-20)

3. Bodyweight Skull Crusher

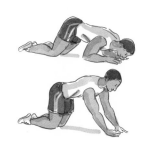

Set 1	Reps: ......13......	(Goal: 10-20)
Set 2	Reps: ......12......	(Goal: 10-20)
Set 3	Reps: ......6......	(Goal: 10-20)
Set 4 (Optional)	Reps: ......5......	(Goal: 10-20)

4. Diamond Push Up

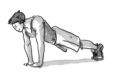

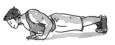

Set 1	Reps: ......7......	(Goal: 10-20)
Set 2	Reps: ......7......	(Goal: 10-20)
Set 3	Reps: ......7......	(Goal: 10-20)
Set 4 (Optional)	Reps: ......6......	(Goal: 10-20)

Supersets Done Today (Circle):

1   2   3   4

Today's Workout Intensity:

8.5 /10

The Three Factors
of Behavior Change

James Clear, author of Atomic Habits, writes that
there are essentially three parts to behavior change
(we love your work, James!).

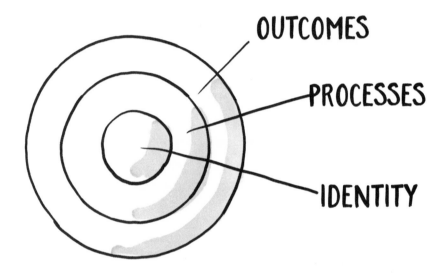

---

1. The Outcomes

The first is the outside layer: The Outcomes. This is synonymous with your
goals. An example of setting your outcomes is:

"I want to reach 15% body fat and have visible abs."

Outcomes are most useful at setting a larger, over-arching vision for
where you want to go. The downsides of over-focusing on your outcomes
are relying on hitting your goals to bring you happiness instead of enjoying
the process, and a lack of practicality for what to do day-to-day.

*Your outcomes are likely to change over the course of your life to match
your ever-evolving goals and needs.*

2. The Processes

The second, middle layer, is about processes — this boils down to what system and action steps you put in place to allow your outcomes to come to fruition. These are things like:

"I will complete my home workout 4 times a week / I will try to increase the reps or difficulty of an exercise each time."

Processes are synonymous with strategies and tactics. These can be very useful, especially when you find one that clicks, and you'll see a number for you to experiment with sprinkled throughout the journal.

These processes are likely to change over time as you test them out.
See what works best for you and switch things up when you get bored / desensitized to them.

3a. Your Identity

This one's the big kahuna. This is the inner-most layer, matching who your internal belief is of yourself as a person. The biggest mistake people make in enacting behavior change is placing way too large of a focus on the first two parts of this puzzle, while entirely forgetting about the third and the most impactful — how you view yourself.

By properly emphasizing WHO you want to grow into, you will maximize your self-respect, satisfaction, and ability to control your actions — more than any motivation or strategy can give you. Your identity is what you can always fall back on to set your intuition, to guide you to what you should really be doing.

An example of setting your identity is:

"I'm someone who does what it takes to get lean, fit, strong, and healthy. I do what's right, not what's easy, in bodyweight training and staying consistent with my nutrition and fitness goals."

*After defining the identity you want to grow into for yourself, chances are this will **not change much**, but rather, only **strengthen over time** based on your actions.*

3b. Your Identity on Your Off-Days

As much as this plays a role in building towards your goals, it's equally as important in regards to times where you fall off the wagon.

Most people subconsciously forget about what their self-identity looks like when this happens, allowing a massive negative self-view to kick in. This leads to a major emotional factor, **guilt**, to kick in, and as many studies have shown, **guilt is a willpower destroyer**.

Instead, mindfully set your identity in these situations...

> *Grow into the person who uses every opportunity of falling off-track to further strengthen your ability to **switch from your off-days back to being on-track**.*

Chances are you won't have perfect consistency with your nutrition and fitness every single day, for the rest of your life, right? Life is about knowing which habits to employ, at the right time, to help you get the most fulfillment out of life.

This involves testing different things and seeing how they serve your life's purpose. In order to really do this, you must master the ability to switch back and forth and discover how to quickly rebuild the momentum you had with your habits, without any guilt that you "lost your mojo."

Be the type of person who can forgive yourself for your mistakes, who will love yourself unconditionally, and be a true best friend to yourself (because if you can't, who will?).

We know these are big emphases on emotional states that can come off as "fluffy," but the truth is our fulfillment in life is directly tied to our emotional states. Learning how to master them is the true feat of this journal, not just building up a specific habit.

Establishing Your Identity

Write your identity statements below.

What kind of person do you want to grow into through this process?

....

....

....

....

....

What kind of person do you want to be when you fall off the wagon of your habits? What do you want to remember about who you are and how you can repurpose these days to serve your life?

....

....

....

....

....

Common Body-Sculpting Myths

You can't build muscle and burn fat at the same time.

Having experienced muscle gain alongside fat loss ourselves, we're happy to say this is false. Look, to build muscle your body has to have energy - we get energy through food. To lose fat, you have to burn energy. When you eat more than you burn, your body stores energy. When you burn more than you eat, your body loses energy.

The point is that your body uses existing fat for energy when you're at a caloric deficit. The energy is there and as long as you're eating enough of the right kinds of protein and carbs, you're protecting your body from burning through muscle as an energy source.

Another point to keep in mind is that although it is possible to have both muscle growth and fat loss occur at the same time, we recommend getting as lean as you'd like FIRST. This can be done via a 10-20% caloric deficit. Afterwards, you can prioritize muscle growth with a slight caloric surplus of roughly 10-20%.

The fastest way to lose fat is cardio.

Easily false. Your diet is the fastest way to lose weight, bar none. Even more importantly, although body-sculpting loses the battle for weight loss against cardio when comparing them minute for minute, body-sculpting will help burn more FAT.

The number on the scale is one thing, but the way you look changes most based on the development of two factors - muscle development and lower body fat.

~~Your genetics determine everything.~~

Definitely not - it's the worst excuse for working on your body and it doesn't make any sense. Of course your bone length, the shape of your body, etc., all play a role in what you CAN look like at your maximum potential. But you can push your body to limits you never thought possible with body-sculpting—you can completely transform the image you have of yourself in your head and in the mirror right now. You can get the body you want, no matter what shape and size you are right now.

~~Women bulk up when they attempt bodyweight exercises.~~

It is REALLY hard to get big. To really grow and look the way you want, you have to work very, very hard. You have to want it for a very long time and work consistently towards it constantly refining as you go through the process.

So, no, performing bodyweight exercises a couple times a week to have adequate, healthy muscle development will not make anybody grow big and bulky.

Falling in *LOVE* with the Process

There is no absolute correct way to work out.

The true secret to strength, muscle growth, and fitness is: you start SOMEWHERE with SOME routine, you stick to it for some time, learn from the experience and move forward from there.

We are giving you a routine that WILL 100% help change your body if you stick to it. But the learning never stops.

We hope this gives you the proper baseline to continue advancing in your body-sculpting goals and strategies so you KEEP getting closer to that dream body.

This whole process is going to be a blast – seriously.

Whether you're experienced in bodyweight exercises or just starting out, we promise, we will help push your boundary constantly. That's what we really fall in love with.

You'll learn about your own psychology...refine your body...grow in strength, size, endurance, and most importantly, you'll feel REALLY good.

You'll find that you regularly just have more energy. You'll consistently get a high from your workouts and you will begin to fall in love with the body in a special way.

The body is our home, the vehicle through which we travel this journey of life. It is infinitely complicated, wonderfully responsive, sensitive, and a primary instrument for inner psychological growth.

Keeping your body in order, inside and out, feels good for a reason.

That good feeling is how you know its importance – almost like how feeling hungry is your signal to eat.

Let's get to it!

Before Starting: Important Things to Keep in Mind for Each Muscle

Back

- Think of your hands as hooks – it's all about pulling. Your hands grip on and your back / lats should be doing all the work to move your body weight.
- When you pull, actively push your chest out and elbows back, allows more of an extension a little more easily.
- Keep your back comfortably straight no matter which workout you're doing. Pulling and winging your back allows you to perform more reps at the expense of form and the best contraction of the muscle you're targeting. You want to avoid this as the contractions are what's important. Proper form leads to the best ones.

Biceps

- Keep your wrists **straight** as if a rod were going from your forearm through your wrist. Don't bend your wrist to ensure that the bicep is the part of the body making the movement.
- Keep your back flat. Maintain a neutral spine position without arcing forwards or backwards.
- Keep your elbows tucked into the body. They should remain still so that your bicep bears the burden of the movement and you're not getting help from the momentum of the rest of the body.
- Remember, the tension is desirable. The contraction is what we want – not just swinging around.
- If you feel you need to lift your elbow upward to finish the movement, your supporting muscles in your forearm are likely too weak – focus on your mind–muscle connection with them.

Chest

- Keep your chest out, traps back, and shoulders down.

Legs

- Number one rule – DO NOT SKIP!
- Whenever you train your legs there will be an increase in your body's testosterone. The more intense your workout is, the more testosterone that's produced. Leg training includes many exercises that work the entire lower portion of the body. As big movements that work many muscles at once, the intensity is very high, producing more testosterone, which benefits all of your growth – upper AND lower body.

Shoulders

- There is a lot of natural swinging that happens when we work shoulders. You have to stay mindful of that and not use momentum for the movement. The whole point is to maximize the muscle contraction, so using the momentum of the swing doesn't do much to help here. Doing 6 good reps is better than 15-20 swinging reps!
- Relax your shoulders and traps, let them fall down and back... and keep them there!

Triceps

- Similar to biceps, keep your wrists STRAIGHT as if a rod were going through your forearm and hand. Don't let your wrist lag back or hold it too tightly forward.
- Keep your elbows tucked inwards to your body to contract as much of the tricep as possible and also hit the lateral head of the tricep.
- Keep your elbows in the same spot as you complete each movement. When your elbows move up and down with the movement, you're compensating with the rest of your upper body and your tricep isn't bearing the entire load.

Note: You will see additional notes & illustrations about improving your form throughout the journal!

General Safety Tips

1. You always want the muscle you're working on...
to take the load, not your back or other parts of the body – all it takes is ONE bad set, ONE bad rep to set you back weeks or even months.

2. Never invent new uses for an exercise!

3. Performing exercises efficiently...
being mindful of not waiting too long between sets is a great thing to do. Performing exercises quickly, sacrificing form and setting yourself up for injury is a really bad idea.

4. Don't extend to the absolute limit of your flexibility...
unless you're extremely comfortable with the exercise.

5. Several exercises have the option...
to utilize a piece of furniture or sturdy object. Please ensure that these are sturdy and the proper height for the exercise.

6. The index has a large amount of exercises...
to use as alternatives if you can't/ are unable/don't want to perform a specific exercise. Use this resource! If in doubt about your safety/ability, swap it out!

7. Always be aware of your surroundings!
Make sure what you're doing doesn't jeopardize anybody else's safety.

8. Always lean on the side of safety...
rather than one of ego or forcing yourself to break personal records. Most importantly, don't do anything that risks injuring yourself, which will set back your progress for a very long time.

9. Pay attention to your past injuries.
If any part of your body is even close to hurting, drastically lower the reps and consider stopping the exercise or workout altogether.

10. Pay close attention to your form.
We give you tips on this throughout the journal and in the index. Good form equals an awesome workout and injury prevention.

Holding Yourself Accountable & Staying Consistent.

One of the best ways to continue doing this habit is to build it alongside a friend who is also passionate about becoming the best version of themself. Having someone to talk to and brainstorm about your specific pain points makes a huge difference. Their support (and sometimes competitive kick) can serve as a nice backup, too.

Whether or not that person is also using this journal alongside you, you're still able to work together on establishing a consistent habit together.

If you're the type of person who benefits from a sense of community, we created a free Facebook group specifically designed to hold yourself accountable to using this journal, getting daily support, and for building habits in general. There's daily activity on there and our team is extremely involved each day.

> Join the Habit Nest accountability group here:
> **facebook.com/groups/habitnest**

Commit.

No matter what happens tomorrow...

Whether I am exhausted
*or have the **worst** day of my life...*

...whether I win the lottery
*Or have the **best** day of my life...*

*I **<u>will</u>** do my workout.*

*My word is like **gold**.*

I will do whatever it takes
to make this happen.

I will workout at least this many times a week (circle one):

1   2   3   4   5   6   7

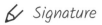 Signature

 Date

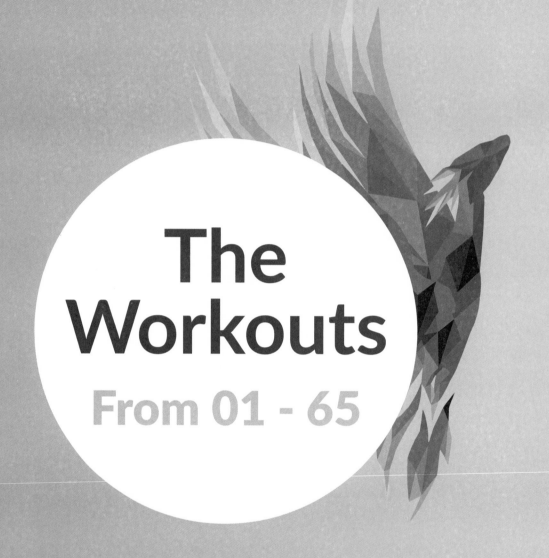

The Workouts

From 01 - 65

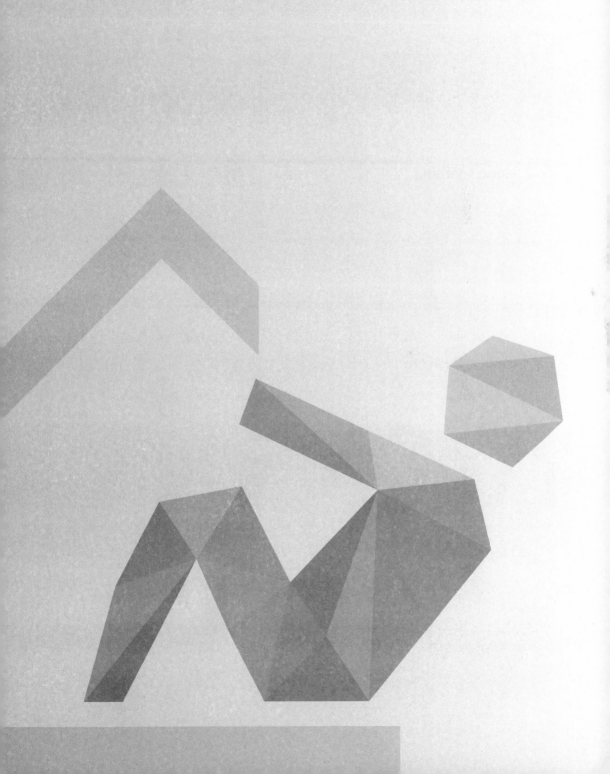

Back & Triceps

Exercise Guide
https://habitnest.link/WGBJ-BW01

(You'll see links to exercise guides here each day.)

1. Simulated Pull Up

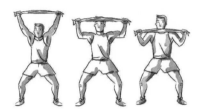

Set 1	Reps: 10	(Goal: 10-20)
Set 2	Reps:	(Goal: 10-20)
Set 3	Reps:	(Goal: 10-20)
Set 4 (Optional)	Reps:	(Goal: 10-20)

2. Good Morning

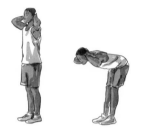

For all exercises, make sure to squeeze the muscles being worked at the climax of the movement and hold for 0.5-1 seconds.

Set 1	Reps: 10	(Goal: 10-20)
Set 2	Reps:	(Goal: 10-20)
Set 3	Reps:	(Goal: 10-20)
Set 4 (Optional)	Reps:	(Goal: 10-20)

3. Scapular Push Up

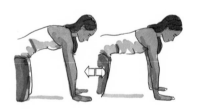

Keep your back straight, not bent forward or backward, to make sure the lats bear the burden of the exercise. Keep your traps fully lowered!

Set 1	Reps: 10	(Goal: 10-20)
Set 2	Reps:	(Goal: 10-20)
Set 3	Reps:	(Goal: 10-20)
Set 4 (Optional)	Reps:	(Goal: 10-20)

4. Doorway Row

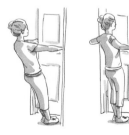

Set 1	Reps: 10	(Goal: 10-20)
Set 2	Reps:	(Goal: 10-20)
Set 3	Reps:	(Goal: 10-20)
Set 4 (Optional)	Reps:	(Goal: 10-20)

Cardio Done Today:

....

Back **& Triceps**

1. Bodyweight Dips

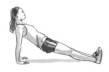

Set 1   Reps: .....10...... (Goal: 10-20)

Set 2   Reps: .... (Goal: 10-20)

Set 3   Reps: .... (Goal: 10-20)

Set 4   Reps: .... (Goal: 10-20)
(Optional)

2. Flexing Overhead Tricep Extension

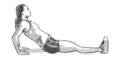

Set 1   Reps: .....10...... (Goal: 10-20)

Set 2   Reps: .... (Goal: 10-20)

Set 3   Reps: .... (Goal: 10-20)

Set 4   Reps: .... (Goal: 10-20)
(Optional)

3. Bodyweight Skull Crusher

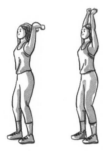

Set 1   Reps: .....10...... (Goal: 10-20)

Set 2   Reps: .... (Goal: 10-20)

Set 3   Reps: .... (Goal: 10-20)

Set 4   Reps: .... (Goal: 10-20)
(Optional)

4. Diamond Push Up

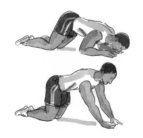

Set 1   Reps: .....X...... (Goal: 10-20)

Set 2   Reps: .... (Goal: 10-20)

Set 3   Reps: .... (Goal: 10-20)

Set 4   Reps: .... (Goal: 10-20)
(Optional)

Supersets consist of doing two exercises back-to-back with no rest in between. Sprinkle them in to speed up your workout and/or add additional challenge!

 Supersets Done Today (Circle):

1   2   3   4

49

 Today's Workout Intensity:

.............../10

Chest & Biceps

Exercise Guide
https://habitnest.link/WGBJ-BW02

1. Stop-and-Release Push Up

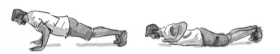

To build some incredible power, after you release your arms up, explode them back down into the floor and push through.

Set 1   Reps: ....   (Goal: 10-20)

Set 2   Reps: ....   (Goal: 10-20)

Set 3   Reps: ....   (Goal: 10-20)

Set 4   Reps: ....   (Goal: 10-20)
(Optional)

2. Decline Prayers

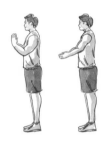

Your goal rest times should be 30-90 seconds between each set/ exercise, including the time it takes you to transition from one exercise to another.

Set 1   Reps: ....   (Goal: 10-20)

Set 2   Reps: ....   (Goal: 10-20)

Set 3   Reps: ....   (Goal: 10-20)

Set 4   Reps: ....   (Goal: 10-20)
(Optional)

3. Incline Push Up

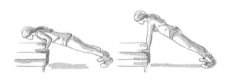

Set 1   Reps: ....   (Goal: 10-20)

Set 2   Reps: ....   (Goal: 10-20)

Set 3   Reps: ....   (Goal: 10-20)

Set 4   Reps: ....   (Goal: 10-20)
(Optional)

4. Prayers

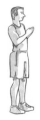
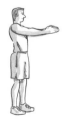

Optional: Hold a flat weight firmly between the palms of your hands!

Set 1   Reps: ....   (Goal: 10-20)

Set 2   Reps: ....   (Goal: 10-20)

Set 3   Reps: ....   (Goal: 10-20)

Set 4   Reps: ....   (Goal: 10-20)
(Optional)

Doing cardio is completely optional. If you do it, use the field on the right to track it using minutes, distance, or whatever metric you prefer.

 Cardio Done Today:

....

Workout 02

Chest **& Biceps**

.........../........../...........
Date

1. Doorway Curl

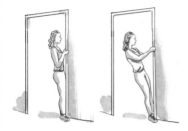

The further you straddle the wall/doorjamb with your legs, the more you'll need to engage your bicep muscles.

Set 1 Reps: .... (Goal: 10-20)

Set 2 Reps: .... (Goal: 10-20)

Set 3 Reps: .... (Goal: 10-20)

Set 4 Reps: .... (Goal: 10-20)
(Optional)

2. Flexing Hammer Curl

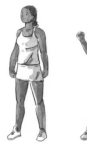
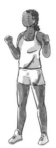

The muscle resistance in this exercise comes from your fists squeezing against themselves. Try to maintain this tension the entire time.

Set 1 Reps: .... (Goal: 10-20)

Set 2 Reps: .... (Goal: 10-20)

Set 3 Reps: .... (Goal: 10-20)

Set 4 Reps: .... (Goal: 10-20)
(Optional)

3. Curl Your Leg

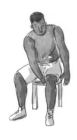
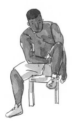

Before you start, ensure that only your buttocks is in contact with the edge of the chair, no thigh-contact.

Set 1 Reps: .... (Goal: 10-20 Each Side)

Set 2 Reps: .... (Goal: 10-20 Each Side)

Set 3 Reps: .... (Goal: 10-20 Each Side)

Set 4 Reps: .... (Goal: 10-20 Each Side)
(Optional)

4. Towel Curl

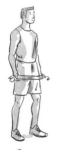
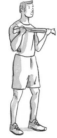

Set 1 Reps: .... (Goal: 10-20)

Set 2 Reps: .... (Goal: 10-20)

Set 3 Reps: .... (Goal: 10-20)

Set 4 Reps: .... (Goal: 10-20)
(Optional)

Supersets Done Today (Circle):

1   2   3   4

Do your best to make each workout at least an 8 in intensity!

 Today's Workout Intensity:

............../10

Legs & Abs

Exercise Guide
https://habitnest.link/WGBJ-BW03

1. Curtsy Lunge

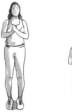

Ensure that your knee doesn't extend beyond your toes.

Set 1 Reps: .... (Goal: 10-20 Each Side)

Set 2 Reps: .... (Goal: 10-20 Each Side)

Set 3 Reps: .... (Goal: 10-20 Each Side)

Set 4 Reps: .... (Goal: 10-20 Each Side)
(Optional)

2. Squat

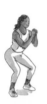

The exercise index at the end of the journal includes detailed workout descriptions for all listed exercises, including 'alternative' ones.

Set 1 Reps: .... (Goal: 10-20)

Set 2 Reps: .... (Goal: 10-20)

Set 3 Reps: .... (Goal: 10-20)

Set 4 Reps: .... (Goal: 10-20)
(Optional)

3. Glute Bridge

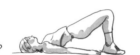

For added difficulty and resistance, you can position a weight or weighted item on your hips and hold it in place as you perform this exercise.

Set 1 Reps: .... (Goal: 10-20)

Set 2 Reps: .... (Goal: 10-20)

Set 3 Reps: .... (Goal: 10-20)

Set 4 Reps: .... (Goal: 10-20)
(Optional)

4. Table + Donkey Kick

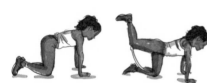

Consider balancing a dumbbell behind your knee or utilizing a resistance band for added challenge.

Set 1 Reps: .... (Goal: 10-20 Each Side)

Set 2 Reps: .... (Goal: 10-20 Each Side)

Set 3 Reps: .... (Goal: 10-20 Each Side)

Set 4 Reps: .... (Goal: 10-20 Each Side)
(Optional)

Variation idea: Do 1/3rd of each set with your toes pointed straight, 1/3rd with your pointed away from each other, and 1/3rd with your toes pointed towards othe

5. Calf Raise

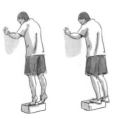

Set 1 Reps: .... (Goal: 10-20)

Set 2 Reps: .... (Goal: 10-20)

Set 3 Reps: .... (Goal: 10-20)

Set 4 Reps: .... (Goal: 10-20)
(Optional)

If you really prefer not to do a given exercise, cross it out and put another in its place!

 Cardio Done Today:

....

Workout 03 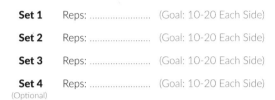 Date: ..../........./............

Legs **& Abs**

1. Spider-Man Plank Crunch

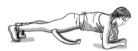
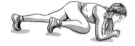

Set 1   Reps: ....   (Goal: 10-20 Each Side)

Set 2   Reps: ....   (Goal: 10-20 Each Side)

Set 3   Reps: ....   (Goal: 10-20 Each Side)

Set 4   Reps: ....   (Goal: 10-20 Each Side)
(Optional)

You'll notice ab exercises only have three sets listed instead of four. This is because the abs are a smaller muscle and are mainly 'made in the kitchen' with good diet, requiring less of an exercise focus on them.

2. Leg Lift

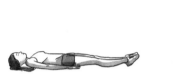

Set 1   Reps: ....   (Goal: 10-20)

Set 2   Reps: ....   (Goal: 10-20)

Set 3   Reps: ....   (Goal: 10-20)

Set 4   Reps: ....   (Goal: 10-20)
(Optional)

3. Starfish Crunch

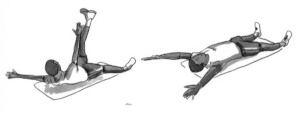

Set 1   Reps: ....   (Goal: 10-20 Each Side)

Set 2   Reps: ....   (Goal: 10-20 Each Side)

Set 3   Reps: ....   (Goal: 10-20 Each Side)

Set 4   Reps: ....   (Goal: 10-20 Each Side)
(Optional)

4. Plank

Make sure to keep your back straight and your abdominal muscles and core locked tight.

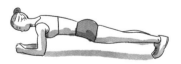

Set 1   Time: ....   (Goal: 45-90 Seconds)

Set 2   Time: ....   (Goal: 45-90 Seconds)

Set 3   Time: ....   (Goal: 45-90 Seconds)

Set 4   Time: ....   (Goal: 45-90 Seconds)
(Optional)

Supersets Done Today (Circle):

1   2   3   4

53

Today's Workout Intensity:

............../10

Shoulders

Exercise Guide
https://habitnest.link/WGBJ-BW04

1. Y Raises

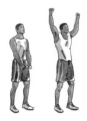

Set 1   Reps: .... (Goal: 10-20)

Set 2   Reps: .... (Goal: 10-20)

Set 3   Reps: .... (Goal: 10-20)

Set 4   Reps: .... (Goal: 10-20)
(Optional)

2. Towel Snatch

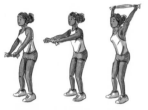

Set 1   Reps: .... (Goal: 10-20)

Set 2   Reps: .... (Goal: 10-20)

Set 3   Reps: .... (Goal: 10-20)

Set 4   Reps: .... (Goal: 10-20)
(Optional)

3. Doorframe Hold

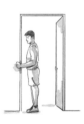

Set 1   Reps: .... (Goal: 10-20 Each Side)

Set 2   Reps: .... (Goal: 10-20 Each Side)

Set 3   Reps: .... (Goal: 10-20 Each Side)

Set 4   Reps: .... (Goal: 10-20 Each Side)
(Optional)

4. Pike Push Up

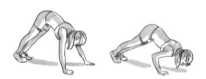

Set 1   Reps: .... (Goal: 10-20)

Set 2   Reps: .... (Goal: 10-20)

Set 3   Reps: .... (Goal: 10-20)

Set 4   Reps: .... (Goal: 10-20)
(Optional)

5. Arm Scissors

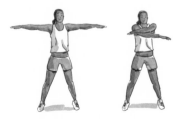

Set 1   Reps: .... (Goal: 10-20)

Set 2   Reps: .... (Goal: 10-20)

Set 3   Reps: .... (Goal: 10-20)

Set 4   Reps: .... (Goal: 10-20)
(Optional)

🏃 Cardio Done Today:

....

6. Reverse Push Up

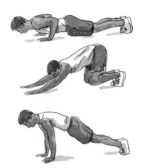

Set 1   Reps: ....   (Goal: 10-20)

Set 2   Reps: ....   (Goal: 10-20)

Set 3   Reps: ....   (Goal: 10-20)

Set 4   Reps: ....   (Goal: 10-20)
(Optional)

7. Side Plank + Twist

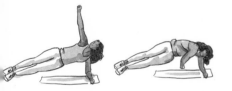

Set 1   Reps: ....   (Goal: 10-20 Each Side)

Set 2   Reps: ....   (Goal: 10-20 Each Side)

Set 3   Reps: ....   (Goal: 10-20 Each Side)

Set 4   Reps: ....   (Goal: 10-20 Each Side)
(Optional)

Full Body Workout

......./......../............
Date

Rest for **15–20 seconds between each exercise**, then rest for **1–2 minutes after completing** the entire circuit. Complete the full circuit **a total of 4–5 times**.

1. Jumping Jacks

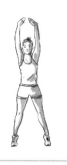

30 seconds

2. Squat

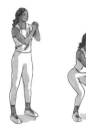

30 seconds

3. Crunch

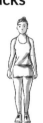

30 seconds

4. Mountain Climber

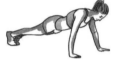
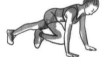

30 seconds

5. Simulated Pull Up

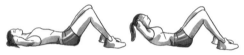
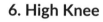

30 seconds

6. High Knee

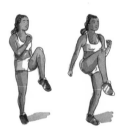

30 seconds

7. In & Out Push-Up

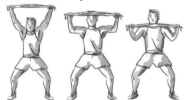

30 seconds

8. Plank

30 seconds

 Circuits Completed (Circle):

1   2   3   4   5

56

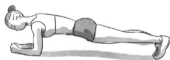 **Today's Workout Intensity:**

................/10

Double Pro-Tip

Create a phone ritual when working out.

When your phone is on and in your pocket as you workout, it's a ticking time bomb of distraction. As Arnold Schwarzenegger stated:

"When I see people texting in the gym, they're not serious. This is Mickey Mouse stuff. You train, or you don't."

You need to conquer your phone and its intensely-distracting-glory at the gym. This works best by creating a ritual with your phone when you arrive.

Aside from being mindful of not using it, you can decrease the amount of distractions it provides by performing the following:

1. Set your phone in airplane mode, or airplane mode and wi-fi on if you're using it to stream music / audiobooks.

2. Turn on "do not disturb" mode.

3. Set your phone to grayscale mode (makes a huge difference). Google how to do this and set it up as a shortcut on your phone.

Set out your workout clothes the night before.

By starting your day with everything you need to get going, you'll feel prepared, organized, and ready to take on your day with momentum!

Packing your gym clothes and bag will help hold you accountable for actually going to the gym that day as well.

This tip is even more effective if you work out early in the mornings as you're able to get up and move!

Psssstt... We like rewarding people (like you) who TAKE ACTION and actually use this journal. Email us now at <u>secret+bodyweight@habitnest.com</u> *for a secret gift ;)*

Back & Triceps

Exercise Guide
https://habitnest.link/WGBJ-BW06

1. Reverse Snow Angel

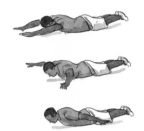

Set 1	Reps:	(Goal: 10-20)
Set 2	Reps:	(Goal: 10-20)
Set 3	Reps:	(Goal: 10-20)
Set 4 (Optional)	Reps:	(Goal: 10-20)

2. Doorway Row

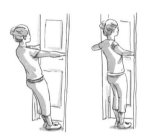

Previous Best (Workout 01)	Reps:	
Set 1	Reps:	(Goal: 10-20)
Set 2	Reps:	(Goal: 10-20)
Set 3	Reps:	(Goal: 10-20)
Set 4 (Optional)	Reps:	(Goal: 10-20)

3. Superman

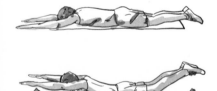

Set 1	Reps:	(Goal: 10-20)
Set 2	Reps:	(Goal: 10-20)
Set 3	Reps:	(Goal: 10-20)
Set 4 (Optional)	Reps:	(Goal: 10-20)

4. Good Morning

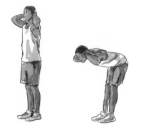

Previous Best (Workout 01)	Reps:	
Set 1	Reps:	(Goal: 10-20)
Set 2	Reps:	(Goal: 10-20)
Set 3	Reps:	(Goal: 10-20)
Set 4 (Optional)	Reps:	(Goal: 10-20)

Cardio Done Today:
....

Back **& Triceps**

1. Y Raises

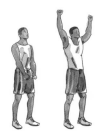

Previous Best
(Workout 04)   Reps: ....

Set 1   Reps: .... (Goal: 10-20)

Set 2   Reps: .... (Goal: 10-20)

Set 3   Reps: .... (Goal: 10-20)

Set 4   Reps: .... (Goal: 10-20)
(Optional)

2. Towel Snatch

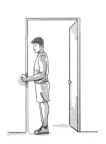

Previous Best
(Workout 04)   Reps: ....

Set 1   Reps: .... (Goal: 10-20)

Set 2   Reps: .... (Goal: 10-20)

Set 3   Reps: .... (Goal: 10-20)

Set 4   Reps: .... (Goal: 10-20)
(Optional)

3. Doorframe Hold

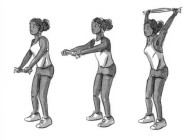

Previous Best
(Workout 04)   Reps: ....

Set 1   Reps: .... (Goal: 10-20 Each Side)

Set 2   Reps: .... (Goal: 10-20 Each Side)

Set 3   Reps: .... (Goal: 10-20 Each Side)

Set 4   Reps: .... (Goal: 10-20 Each Side)
(Optional)

4. Side Plank + Twist

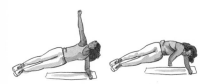

Previous Best
(Workout 04)   Reps: ....

Set 1   Reps: .... (Goal: 10-20 Each Side)

Set 2   Reps: .... (Goal: 10-20 Each Side)

Set 3   Reps: .... (Goal: 10-20 Each Side)

Set 4   Reps: .... (Goal: 10-20 Each Side)
(Optional)

Supersets Done Today (Circle):

1   2   3   4

Today's Workout Intensity:

.............../10

Push Up

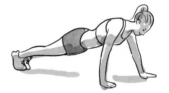

Problem

You don't perform the full range of motion.

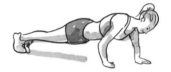

Improper form

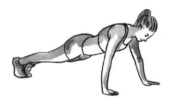

How to Fix This

Avoid performing push ups too quickly; give yourself time to get into proper position and in a slow, controlled fashion, lower yourself downward until your chest comes as close as possible to the ground before engaging your chest muscles and pushing back up.

Consider recording yourself performing pushups (and other exercises) so you can **evaluate your form.**

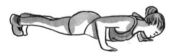

Proper form

Flexing Exercises

Problem

You aren't engaging your muscles properly.

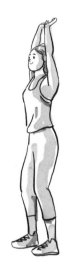

Improper form

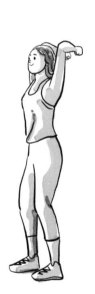
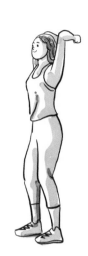

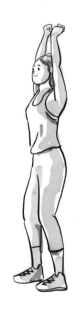

How to Fix This

For flexing exercises, the resistance comes from your own fist. Imagine you are trying to push your fingers through the other side of your hand while performing these exercises.

Proper form

Biceps & Triceps

1. Doorway Curl

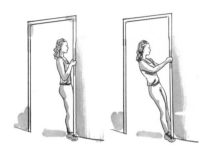

Previous Best
(Workout 02)   Reps: ....

Set 1   Reps: .... (Goal: 10-20)

Set 2   Reps: .... (Goal: 10-20)

Set 3   Reps: .... (Goal: 10-20)

Set 4
(Optional)   Reps: .... (Goal: 10-20)

2. Flexing Hammer Curl

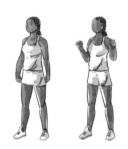

Previous Best
(Workout 02)   Reps: ....

Set 1   Reps: .... (Goal: 10-20)

Set 2   Reps: .... (Goal: 10-20)

Set 3   Reps: .... (Goal: 10-20)

Set 4
(Optional)   Reps: .... (Goal: 10-20)

3. Towel Curl

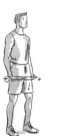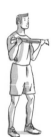

Previous Best
(Workout 02)   Reps: ....

Set 1   Reps: .... (Goal: 10-20)

Set 2   Reps: .... (Goal: 10-20)

Set 3   Reps: .... (Goal: 10-20)

Set 4
(Optional)   Reps: .... (Goal: 10-20)

4. Side Laying Bicep Curl

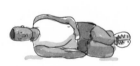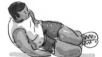

Set 1   Reps: .... (Goal: 10-20)

Set 2   Reps: .... (Goal: 10-20)

Set 3   Reps: .... (Goal: 10-20)

Set 4
(Optional)   Reps: .... (Goal: 10-20)

Cardio Done Today:

....

Biceps **& Triceps**

1. Bodyweight Dips

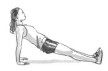
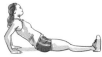

Previous Best Reps: ....
(Workout 01)

Set 1 Reps: .... (Goal: 10-20)

Set 2 Reps: .... (Goal: 10-20)

Set 3 Reps: .... (Goal: 10-20)

Set 4 Reps: .... (Goal: 10-20)
(Optional)

2. Flexing Overhead Tricep Extension

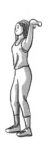
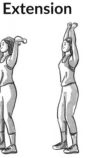

Previous Best Reps: ....
(Workout 01)

Set 1 Reps: .... (Goal: 10-20)

Set 2 Reps: .... (Goal: 10-20)

Set 3 Reps: .... (Goal: 10-20)

Set 4 Reps: .... (Goal: 10-20)
(Optional)

3. Bodyweight Skull Crusher

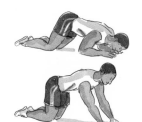

Previous Best Reps: ....
(Workout 01)

Set 1 Reps: .... (Goal: 10-20)

Set 2 Reps: .... (Goal: 10-20)

Set 3 Reps: .... (Goal: 10-20)

Set 4 Reps: .... (Goal: 10-20)
(Optional)

4. Diamond Push Up

Previous Best Reps: ....
(Workout 01)

Set 1 Reps: .... (Goal: 10-20)

Set 2 Reps: .... (Goal: 10-20)

Set 3 Reps: .... (Goal: 10-20)

Set 4 Reps: .... (Goal: 10-20)
(Optional)

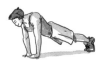 **Supersets Done Today (Circle):**

1   2   3   4

 Today's Workout Intensity:

.............../10

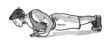

Chest

Exercise Guide
https://habitnest.link/WGBJ-BW08

*For best results, do all exercises,
especially push ups, to failure.*

1. Stop-and-Release Push Up

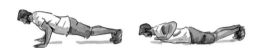

Previous Best (Workout 02)	Reps:	
Set 1	Reps:	(Goal: 10-20)
Set 2	Reps:	(Goal: 10-20)
Set 3	Reps:	(Goal: 10-20)
Set 4 (Optional)	Reps:	(Goal: 10-20)

*The resistance and muscle work here is centered
on your hands pushing against each other. Keep
that tension throughout the movement.*

2. Decline Prayers

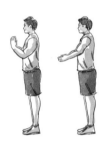

Previous Best (Workout 02)	Reps:	
Set 1	Reps:	(Goal: 10-20)
Set 2	Reps:	(Goal: 10-20)
Set 3	Reps:	(Goal: 10-20)
Set 4 (Optional)	Reps:	(Goal: 10-20)

*Try out different heights to incline your push up and see
which gives you your best challenge, without losing form.*

3. Incline Push Up

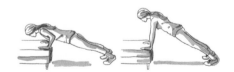

Previous Best (Workout 02)	Reps:	
Set 1	Reps:	(Goal: 10-20)
Set 2	Reps:	(Goal: 10-20)
Set 3	Reps:	(Goal: 10-20)
Set 4 (Optional)	Reps:	(Goal: 10-20)

Cardio Done Today:

....

Chest

4. Push Up

Even if you have past experience doing these exercises, that doesn't necessarily mean they've been done correctly. We cover the little nuances with each exercise that separates good from bad form in the index - we recommend reading the whole thing.

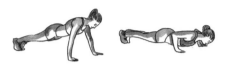

Set 1 Reps: .... (Goal: 10-20)

Set 2 Reps: .... (Goal: 10-20)

Set 3 Reps: .... (Goal: 10-20)

Set 4 Reps: .... (Goal: 10-20)
(Optional)

5. In & Out Push Up

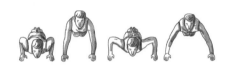

Set 1 Reps: .... (Goal: 10-20)

Set 2 Reps: .... (Goal: 10-20)

Set 3 Reps: .... (Goal: 10-20)

Set 4 Reps: .... (Goal: 10-20)
(Optional)

6. Incline Prayers

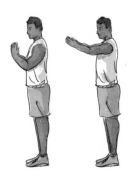

Set 1 Reps: .... (Goal: 10-20)

Set 2 Reps: .... (Goal: 10-20)

Set 3 Reps: .... (Goal: 10-20)

Set 4 Reps: .... (Goal: 10-20)
(Optional)

Supersets Done Today (Circle):

1   2   3   4

Today's Workout Intensity:

................/10

Legs & Abs

1. Bodyweight Deadlift

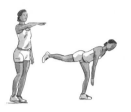

As you encounter new exercises in the journal, experiment with different, safe rep ranges to learn what works best for you over time.

Set 1 Reps: .... (Goal: 10-20 Each Side)

Set 2 Reps: .... (Goal: 10-20 Each Side)

Set 3 Reps: .... (Goal: 10-20 Each Side)

Set 4 Reps: .... (Goal: 10-20 Each Side)
(Optional)

2. Curtsy Lunge

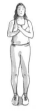

Previous Best Reps: ....
(Workout 03)

Set 1 Reps: .... (Goal: 10-20 Each Side)

Set 2 Reps: .... (Goal: 10-20 Each Side)

Set 3 Reps: .... (Goal: 10-20 Each Side)

Set 4 Reps: .... (Goal: 10-20 Each Side)
(Optional)

Really focus on squeezing those glute muscles at the top of this movement!

3. Glute Bridge

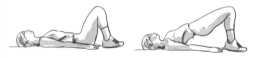

Previous Best Reps: ....
(Workout 03)

Set 1 Reps: .... (Goal: 10-20)

Set 2 Reps: .... (Goal: 10-20)

Set 3 Reps: .... (Goal: 10-20)

Set 4 Reps: .... (Goal: 10-20)
(Optional)

4. Table + Donkey Kick

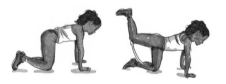

Previous Best Reps: ....
(Workout 03)

Set 1 Reps: .... (Goal: 10-20 Each Side)

Set 2 Reps: .... (Goal: 10-20 Each Side)

Set 3 Reps: .... (Goal: 10-20 Each Side)

Set 4 Reps: .... (Goal: 10-20 Each Side)
(Optional)

5. Calf Raise

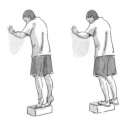

Previous Best Reps: ....
(Workout 03)

Set 1 Reps: .... (Goal: 10-20)

Set 2 Reps: .... (Goal: 10-20)

Set 3 Reps: .... (Goal: 10-20)

Set 4 Reps: .... (Goal: 10-20)
(Optional)

Cardio Done Today:

....

Legs **& Abs**

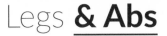

1. Spider-Man Plank Crunch

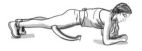
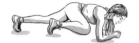

Previous Best
(Workout 03)   Reps: ....

Set 1   Reps: ....   (Goal: 10-20 Each Side)

Set 2   Reps: ....   (Goal: 10-20 Each Side)

Set 3   Reps: ....   (Goal: 10-20 Each Side)

Set 4   Reps: ....   (Goal: 10-20 Each Side)
(Optional)

2. Leg Lift

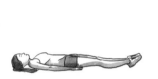

Previous Best
(Workout 03)   Reps: ....

Set 1   Reps: ....   (Goal: 10-20)

Set 2   Reps: ....   (Goal: 10-20)

Set 3   Reps: ....   (Goal: 10-20)

Set 4   Reps: ....   (Goal: 10-20)
(Optional)

Filling out the 'Previous Best' section is very important, as it sets a clear goal for you to beat and lets you see the progress you're making after each workout.

3. Starfish Crunch

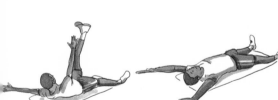

Previous Best
(Workout 03)   Reps: ....

Set 1   Reps: ....   (Goal: 10-20 Each Side)

Set 2   Reps: ....   (Goal: 10-20 Each Side)

Set 3   Reps: ....   (Goal: 10-20 Each Side)

Set 4   Reps: ....   (Goal: 10-20 Each Side)
(Optional)

4. Plank

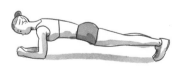

Previous Best
(Workout 03)   Reps: ....

Set 1   Time: ....   (Goal: 45-90 Seconds)

Set 2   Time: ....   (Goal: 45-90 Seconds)

Set 3   Time: ....   (Goal: 45-90 Seconds)

Set 4   Time: ....   (Goal: 45-90 Seconds)
(Optional)

Supersets Done Today (Circle):

1   2   3   4

Today's Workout Intensity:

................/10

Full Body Workout

........./........./...........
Date

Rest for **15–20 seconds between each exercise**, then rest for **1–2 minutes after completing** the entire circuit. Complete the full circuit **a total of 4–5 times**.

1. Run In Place

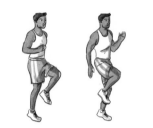

30 seconds

2. Alternating Lunge

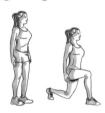

30 seconds

3. Starfish Crunch

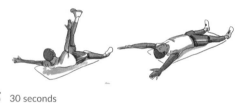

30 seconds

4. Towel Snatch

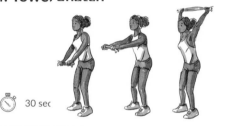

30 sec

5. Push Up

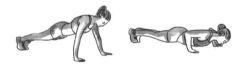

30 seconds

6. High Knee

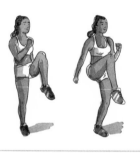

30 seconds

7. Burpee

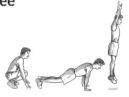

30 seconds

8. Bicycle Crunch

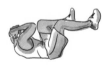
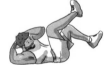

30 seconds

Circuits Completed (Circle):

1   2   3   4   5

68

Today's Workout Intensity:

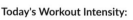

.............../10

Check-In

Taking a few minutes to simply STOP and evaluate how you're doing mentally, physically, and emotionally every few weeks of a training program can be extremely helpful to your experience with it.

Take a few minutes to answer the following questions with honesty!

What do I expect out of this process? How do I want to look? Feel?

....

....

....

How am I feeling about the quality and intensity of my workouts?

....

....

....

How do I feel about the way I look?

....

....

....

What do I want to learn more about (e.g. muscle anatomy, nutrition, mobility, etc.) that I can spend some time researching?

....

....

....

Bonus Challenge

> *Achieve a deep*
> *mind-muscle connection*
> *with every single rep you perform.*

We talked about the scientific importance of having mind-muscle connection in the intro of this journal, but it is so imperative (and so easy to misunderstand) that it's worth repeating here.

Many people understand mind-muscle connection as simply 'being focused' and 'not being distracted' during workouts. Although that's part of it, the true effectiveness of mind-muscle connection comes when you:

1. Turn off all other muscles that are not part of the movement. Only lift/use the bodyweight with the specific muscles needed for it.

2. Keep the muscle(s) you're using fully engaged, flexed, and isolated the entire time throughout each movement. For every second of every rep.

To take this concept to the next level, you should isolate and flex the specific muscle you're going to use before every single exercise so you'll know exactly what to activate with each rep.

This means at the top or bottom of each rep, you keep your muscle engaged and fully lifting your bodyweight as you would in the middle of a rep.

You may have to drastically drop in reps to do this, which is a sign you're doing a substantial amount of 'cheating reps' and leaving lots of a movement's primary muscles barely used.

You should also be prepared to know what muscles can help you break form and cheat so you can be extra vigilant of not using them.

Play around with this concept during your next workout if it's new for you and see if you notice a big difference.

Back & Abs

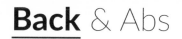

Fun Fact: Bodyweight exercises allow you to work on and perfect your form f
when you perform these same exercises at the gym, with weights.

1. Simulated Pull Up

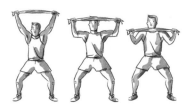

Previous Best (Workout 01)	Reps:	
Set 1	Reps:	(Goal: 10-20)
Set 2	Reps:	(Goal: 10-20)
Set 3	Reps:	(Goal: 10-20)
Set 4 (Optional)	Reps:	(Goal: 10-20)

Note: You'll never fully feel ready to add challenge to
an exercise. Try to challenge yourself anyway.

2. Doorway Row

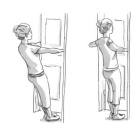

Previous Best (Workout 06)	Reps:	
Set 1	Reps:	(Goal: 10-20)
Set 2	Reps:	(Goal: 10-20)
Set 3	Reps:	(Goal: 10-20)
Set 4 (Optional)	Reps:	(Goal: 10-20)

3. Superman

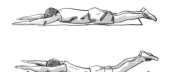

Previous Best (Workout 06)	Reps:	
Set 1	Reps:	(Goal: 10-20)
Set 2	Reps:	(Goal: 10-20)
Set 3	Reps:	(Goal: 10-20)
Set 4 (Optional)	Reps:	(Goal: 10-20)

4. Scapular Push Up

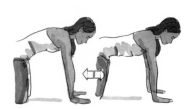

Previous Best (Workout 01)	Reps:	
Set 1	Reps:	(Goal: 10-20)
Set 2	Reps:	(Goal: 10-20)
Set 3	Reps:	(Goal: 10-20)
Set 4 (Optional)	Reps:	(Goal: 10-20)

Cardio Done Today:

....

Back **& Abs**

1. Spider-Man Plank Crunch

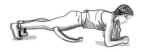

Previous Best   Reps: ....
(Workout 09)

Set 1   Reps: ....   (Goal: 10-20 Each Side)

Set 2   Reps: ....   (Goal: 10-20 Each Side)

Set 3   Reps: ....   (Goal: 10-20 Each Side)

Set 4   Reps: ....   (Goal: 10-20 Each Side)
(Optional)

2. Leg Lift

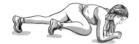

Previous Best   Reps: ....
(Workout 09)

Set 1   Reps: ....   (Goal: 10-20)

Set 2   Reps: ....   (Goal: 10-20)

Set 3   Reps: ....   (Goal: 10-20)

Set 4   Reps: ....   (Goal: 10-20)
(Optional)

You don't have to wait until you feel ready to begin each new set. Try starting sets even when it doesn't feel naturally right to push yourself and maintain a high level of intensity.

3. Russian Twist

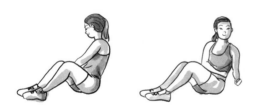

Set 1   Reps: ....   (Goal: 10-20 Each Side)

Set 2   Reps: ....   (Goal: 10-20 Each Side)

Set 3   Reps: ....   (Goal: 10-20 Each Side)

Set 4   Reps: ....   (Goal: 10-20 Each Side)
(Optional)

4. Plank

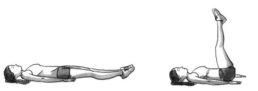

Previous Best   Reps: ....
(Workout 09)

Set 1   Time: ....   (Goal: 45-90 Seconds)

Set 2   Time: ....   (Goal: 45-90 Seconds)

Set 3   Time: ....   (Goal: 45-90 Seconds)

Set 4   Time: ....   (Goal: 45-90 Seconds)
(Optional)

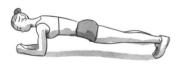

Supersets Done Today (Circle):

1   2   3   4

Today's Workout Intensity:

.............../10

Push Up

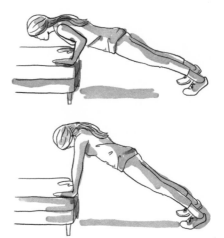

Problem

You dip your head while performing a push up.

Improper form

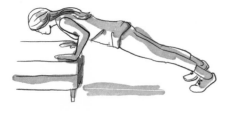

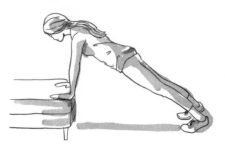

How to Fix This

As you get into position for your push up, pay close attention to your body line. You should be able to draw a straight line from the tip of your head to your heels and maintain this throughout the exercise. If you find your head sagging downward, you may be performing more reps than you're capable of. More reps is good, but only if you're doing them properly.

Proper form

Doorway Exercises

Problem

The exercise feels too easy.

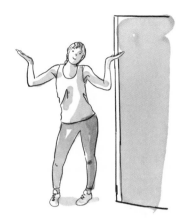

Improper form

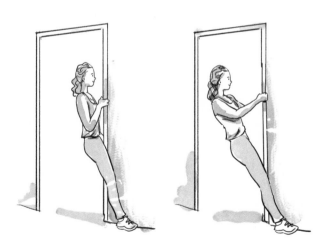

Proper form

How to Fix This

Increase the difficulty of these exercises by stepping through the doorway (for Doorway Rows) or straddling the wall/doorjamb with feet on either side. Experiment with different angles to create more challenge.

Chest & Biceps

Exercise Guide
https://habitnest.link/WGBJ-BW12

1. Stop-and-Release Push Up

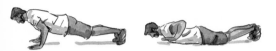

Previous Best
(Workout 08)   Reps: ....

Set 1	Reps:	(Goal: 10-20)
Set 2	Reps:	(Goal: 10-20)
Set 3	Reps:	(Goal: 10-20)
Set 4 (Optional)	Reps:	(Goal: 10-20)

2. Decline Prayers

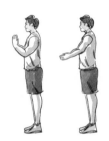

Previous Best
(Workout 08)   Reps: ....

Set 1	Reps:	(Goal: 10-20)
Set 2	Reps:	(Goal: 10-20)
Set 3	Reps:	(Goal: 10-20)
Set 4 (Optional)	Reps:	(Goal: 10-20)

3. Incline Push Up

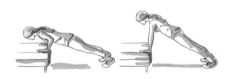

Previous Best
(Workout 08)   Reps: ....

Set 1	Reps:	(Goal: 10-20)
Set 2	Reps:	(Goal: 10-20)
Set 3	Reps:	(Goal: 10-20)
Set 4 (Optional)	Reps:	(Goal: 10-20)

Be very careful performing this exercise. Be sure to have a sturdy piece of furniture and if you're at all concerned for your safety or ability to perform this, please substitute a different exercise.

4. Decline Push Up

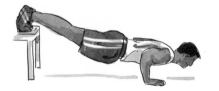

Previous Best
(Workout 08)   Reps: ....

Set 1	Reps:	(Goal: 10-20)
Set 2	Reps:	(Goal: 10-20)
Set 3	Reps:	(Goal: 10-20)
Set 4 (Optional)	Reps:	(Goal: 10-20)

Cardio Done Today:

....

Chest **& Biceps**

1. Doorway Curl

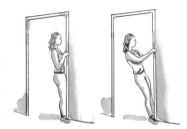

Previous Best
(Workout 07)   Reps: ....

Set 1   Reps: ....   (Goal: 10-20)

Set 2   Reps: ....   (Goal: 10-20)

Set 3   Reps: ....   (Goal: 10-20)

Set 4   Reps: ....   (Goal: 10-20)
(Optional)

2. Towel Curl

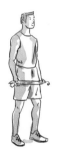
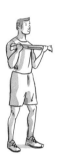

Previous Best
(Workout 07)   Reps: ....

Set 1   Reps: ....   (Goal: 10-20)

Set 2   Reps: ....   (Goal: 10-20)

Set 3   Reps: ....   (Goal: 10-20)

Set 4   Reps: ....   (Goal: 10-20)
(Optional)

*Squeeze and hold for 0.5-1 seconds at the climax
of the movement — when your arms straighten out.*

3. Flexing Hammer Curl

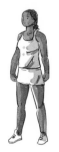
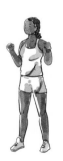

Previous Best
(Workout 07)   Reps: ....

Set 1   Reps: ....   (Goal: 10-20)

Set 2   Reps: ....   (Goal: 10-20)

Set 3   Reps: ....   (Goal: 10-20)

Set 4   Reps: ....   (Goal: 10-20)
(Optional)

4. Curl Your Leg

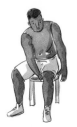
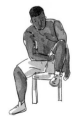

Previous Best
(Workout 02)   Reps: ....

Set 1   Reps: ....   (Goal: 10-20 Each Side)

Set 2   Reps: ....   (Goal: 10-20 Each Side)

Set 3   Reps: ....   (Goal: 10-20 Each Side)

Set 4   Reps: ....   (Goal: 10-20 Each Side)
(Optional)

Supersets Done Today (Circle):

1   2   3   4

Today's Workout Intensity:

............../10

Triceps & Shoulders

1. Bodyweight Dips

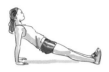
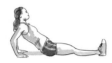

Previous Best
(Workout 07)   Reps: ....

Set 1   Reps: ....   (Goal: 10-20)

Set 2   Reps: ....   (Goal: 10-20)

Set 3   Reps: ....   (Goal: 10-20)

Set 4   Reps: ....   (Goal: 10-20)
(Optional)

2. Flexing Overhead Tricep Extension

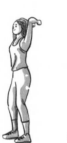
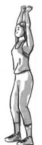

Previous Best
(Workout 07)   Reps: ....

Set 1   Reps: ....   (Goal: 10-20)

Set 2   Reps: ....   (Goal: 10-20)

Set 3   Reps: ....   (Goal: 10-20)

Set 4   Reps: ....   (Goal: 10-20)
(Optional)

If you have trouble, you can do this on your knees.

3. Diamond Push Up

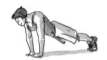
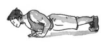

Previous Best
(Workout 07)   Reps: ....

Set 1   Reps: ....   (Goal: 10-20)

Set 2   Reps: ....   (Goal: 10-20)

Set 3   Reps: ....   (Goal: 10-20)

Set 4   Reps: ....   (Goal: 10-20)
(Optional)

4. Bodyweight Skull Crusher

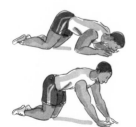

Previous Best
(Workout 07)   Reps: ....

Set 1   Reps: ....   (Goal: 10-20)

Set 2   Reps: ....   (Goal: 10-20)

Set 3   Reps: ....   (Goal: 10-20)

Set 4   Reps: ....   (Goal: 10-20)
(Optional)

Cardio Done Today:

....

Workout 13   Triceps **& Shoulders**

........./........./...........
Date

1. Pike Push Up

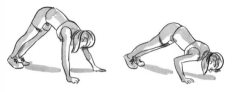

You do not want your head to go straight down in this move. Your head should go forward as you lower down.

Previous Best
(Workout 04)   Reps: ....

Set 1   Reps: ....   (Goal: 10-20)

Set 2   Reps: ....   (Goal: 10-20)

Set 3   Reps: ....   (Goal: 10-20)

Set 4   Reps: ....   (Goal: 10-20)
(Optional)

2. Y Raises

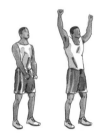

Try not to swing your arms throughout the movement.

Previous Best
(Workout 06)   Reps: ....

Set 1   Reps: ....   (Goal: 10-20)

Set 2   Reps: ....   (Goal: 10-20)

Set 3   Reps: ....   (Goal: 10-20)

Set 4   Reps: ....   (Goal: 10-20)
(Optional)

3. Towel Snatch

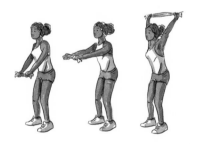

Previous Best
(Workout 06)   Reps: ....

Set 1   Reps: ....   (Goal: 10-20)

Set 2   Reps: ....   (Goal: 10-20)

Set 3   Reps: ....   (Goal: 10-20)

Set 4   Reps: ....   (Goal: 10-20)
(Optional)

4. Side Plank + Twist

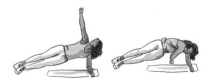

Previous Best
(Workout 06)   Reps: ....

Set 1   Reps: ....   (Goal: 10-20 Each Side)

Set 2   Reps: ....   (Goal: 10-20 Each Side)

Set 3   Reps: ....   (Goal: 10-20 Each Side)

Set 4   Reps: ....   (Goal: 10-20 Each Side)
(Optional)

Supersets Done Today (Circle):

1   2   3   4

 Today's Workout Intensity:

.............../10

Legs

Problem

You're skipping legs day.

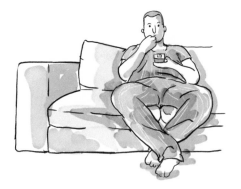

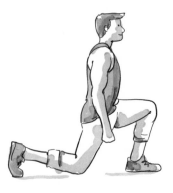

How to Fix This

Understand that legs day will drastically boost your testosterone and help fuel muscle growth for other muscles.

Also, if you work your legs to the limit, they'll grow more quickly than the rest of the body. It can both serve as a good confidence boost and signal that you're moving in the right direction with your training.

Abs

Problem

You're overly relying on ab exercises to get visible abs.

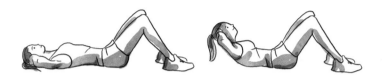

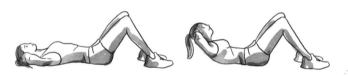

+

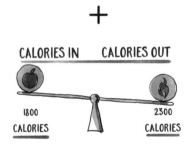

CALORIES IN   CALORIES OUT

1800 CALORIES   2300 CALORIES

How to Fix This

Strengthening your abs, obliques, and core has its benefits (e.g. improving posture, allowing you to lift more in other movements, etc.) but is not enough alone to visibly define your abs.
The main determinate of visible abs is going to be a low body fat % (10% or below for males, 15-20% or below for females).

81

Legs & Abs

1. Bodyweight Deadlift

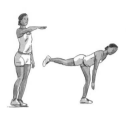

Previous Best (Workout 09) — Reps: ....

Set 1	Reps:	(Goal: 10-20 Each Side)
Set 2	Reps:	(Goal: 10-20 Each Side)
Set 3	Reps:	(Goal: 10-20 Each Side)
Set 4 (Optional)	Reps:	(Goal: 10-20 Each Side)

2. Squat

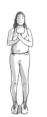 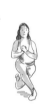

Reminder: If you feel pain with any exercise, STOP! Do NOT push through. Try a different exercise instead.

Previous Best (Workout 03) — Reps: ....

Set 1	Reps:	(Goal: 10-20)
Set 2	Reps:	(Goal: 10-20)
Set 3	Reps:	(Goal: 10-20)
Set 4 (Optional)	Reps:	(Goal: 10-20)

Make sure your knees don't pass your toes when the step is taken! The goal is to go as straight down as possible.

3. Curtsy Lunge

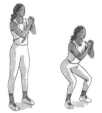

Previous Best (Workout 09) — Reps: ....

Set 1	Reps:	(Goal: 10-20 Each Side)
Set 2	Reps:	(Goal: 10-20 Each Side)
Set 3	Reps:	(Goal: 10-20 Each Side)
Set 4 (Optional)	Reps:	(Goal: 10-20 Each Side)

4. Vertical Leap

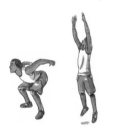

Set 1	Reps:	(Goal: 10-20)
Set 2	Reps:	(Goal: 10-20)
Set 3	Reps:	(Goal: 10-20)
Set 4 (Optional)	Reps:	(Goal: 10-20)

5. Calf Raise

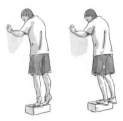

Previous Best (Workout 09) — Reps: ....

Set 1	Reps:	(Goal: 10-20)
Set 2	Reps:	(Goal: 10-20)
Set 3	Reps:	(Goal: 10-20)
Set 4 (Optional)	Reps:	(Goal: 10-20)

Cardio Done Today:

....

Legs **& Abs**

1. Spider-Man Plank Crunch

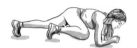
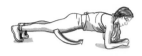

Previous Best
(Workout 11)

Reps: ....

You'll notice ab exercises only have three sets listed instead of four. This is because the abs are a smaller muscle and are mainly 'made in the kitchen' with good diet, requiring less of an exercise focus on them.

2. Leg Lift

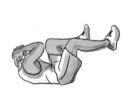

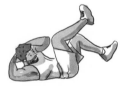

Previous Best
(Workout 11)

Reps: ....

Set 1	Reps:	(Goal: 10-20)
Set 2	Reps:	(Goal: 10-20)
Set 3	Reps:	(Goal: 10-20)
Set 4 (Optional)	Reps:	(Goal: 10-20)

3. Bicycle Crunch

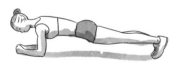

Previous Best
(Workout 09)

Reps: ....

Set 1	Reps:	(Goal: 10-20 Each Side)
Set 2	Reps:	(Goal: 10-20 Each Side)
Set 3	Reps:	(Goal: 10-20 Each Side)
Set 4 (Optional)	Reps:	(Goal: 10-20 Each Side)

Make sure to keep your back straight and your abdominal muscles and core locked tight.

4. Plank

Previous Best
(Workout 11)

Reps: ....

Set 1	Time:	(Goal: 45-90 Seconds)
Set 2	Time:	(Goal: 45-90 Seconds)
Set 3	Time:	(Goal: 45-90 Seconds)
Set 4 (Optional)	Time:	(Goal: 45-90 Seconds)

Supersets Done Today (Circle):

1   2   3   4

83

 Today's Workout Intensity:

............../10

Full Body Workout

Exercise Guide
https://habitnest.link/WGBJ-BW15

Rest for **15–20 seconds between each exercise**, then rest for **1–2 minutes after completing** the entire circuit. Complete the full circuit **a total of 4–5 times**.

1. Jump

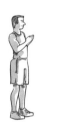
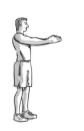

30 seconds

2. Simulated Pull Up

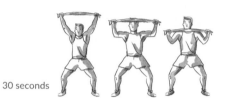

30 seconds

3. Prayers

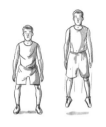

30 seconds

4. Side Plank

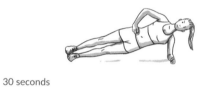

30 seconds

5. Crunch

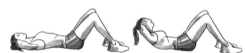
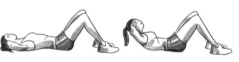

30 seconds

6. High Knee

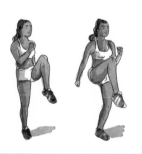

30 seconds

7. Squat

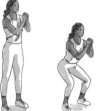

30 seconds

8. Side Plank

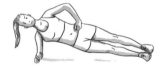

30 seconds

 Circuits Completed (Circle):

1   2   3   4   5

84

 Today's Workout Intensity:

................/10

Pro-Tip

> *Push for progressive overload*
> *week after week.*

You can achieve a new level of progressive overload in 3 different ways:

1. Add resistance bands/weights to your bodyweight work out,

2. Increase the reps you do, or

3. Increase the speed/intensity you complete the workout in.

You have to hit progressive overload in at least one of these ways in order to build more muscle and grow stronger.

One effective way to build this as a habit is by doing one extra rep at the end of each set once you feel you've 'really hit failure.'

If you fail and can't do that extra rep, try holding / supporting the movement for as long as possible, even if it's a half-rep (and make sure it's safe to do so without injuring yourself).

This will give you a crazy additional pump.

If you DO end up completing that additional rep, that's a huge win, as you're breaking into new levels of intensity.

You'll also be learning that you may have extra fuel in the tank to push your workouts even harder. If you end up completing this extra rep, keep going to see if you can complete even more afterwards.

Push yourself and your body to go further throughout the remainder of this journal.

Be safe. Push yourself.

Triceps & Biceps

Exercise Guide
https://habitnest.link/WGBJ-BW16

1. Bodyweight Dips

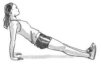

This can also be performed by resting your hands on the edge of a sturdy piece of furniture or box.

Previous Best
(Workout 13)   Reps: ....

Set 1   Reps: ....   (Goal: 10-20)

Set 2   Reps: ....   (Goal: 10-20)

Set 3   Reps: ....   (Goal: 10-20)

Set 4   Reps: ....   (Goal: 10-20)
(Optional)

2. Flexing Overhead Tricep Extension

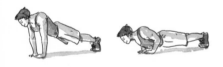

Feel free to add in descriptive notes for yourself to keep in mind, e.g. 'too easy' or 'too heavy' for the exercises. This can help you choose whether to increase reps or utilize a more challenging variation of the exercise.

Previous Best
(Workout 13)   Reps: ....

Set 1   Reps: ....   (Goal: 10-20)

Set 2   Reps: ....   (Goal: 10-20)

Set 3   Reps: ....   (Goal: 10-20)

Set 4   Reps: ....   (Goal: 10-20)
(Optional)

3. Diamond Push Up

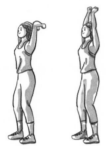

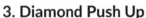

This exercise can also be performed with your hands resting on a sturdy bench or other elevated surface. Keep your back straight, lower your head below your triceps, then bring yourself back up.

Previous Best
(Workout 13)   Reps: ....

Set 1   Reps: ....   (Goal: 10-20)

Set 2   Reps: ....   (Goal: 10-20)

Set 3   Reps: ....   (Goal: 10-20)

Set 4   Reps: ....   (Goal: 10-20)
(Optional)

4. Bodyweight Skull Crusher

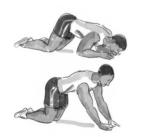

Make sure to move slower on the way down and faster on the way up.

Previous Best
(Workout 13)   Reps: ....

Set 1   Reps: ....   (Goal: 10-20)

Set 2   Reps: ....   (Goal: 10-20)

Set 3   Reps: ....   (Goal: 10-20)

Set 4   Reps: ....   (Goal: 10-20)
(Optional)

Cardio Done Today:

....

Triceps **& Biceps**

1. Curl Your Leg

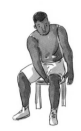
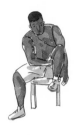

Previous Best
(Workout 12)   Reps: ....

Set 1   Reps: ....   (Goal: 10-20 Each Side)

Set 2   Reps: ....   (Goal: 10-20 Each Side)

Set 3   Reps: ....   (Goal: 10-20 Each Side)

Set 4   Reps: ....   (Goal: 10-20 Each Side)
(Optional)

Mixing a pull-muscle (back) with a push-muscle (triceps) is intended and will help engage multiple parts of your body together.

2. Flexing Hammer Curl

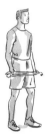
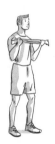

Previous Best
(Workout 12)   Reps: ....

Set 1   Reps: ....   (Goal: 10-20)

Set 2   Reps: ....   (Goal: 10-20)

Set 3   Reps: ....   (Goal: 10-20)

Set 4   Reps: ....   (Goal: 10-20)
(Optional)

Squeeze and hold for 0.5-1 seconds at the climax of the movement — when your arms straighten out.

3. Towel Curl

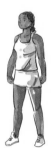
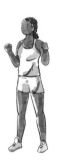

Previous Best
(Workout 12)   Reps: ....

Set 1   Reps: ....   (Goal: 10-20)

Set 2   Reps: ....   (Goal: 10-20)

Set 3   Reps: ....   (Goal: 10-20)

Set 4   Reps: ....   (Goal: 10-20)
(Optional)

4. Flexing Curl

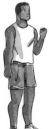
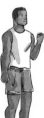
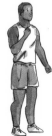
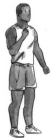

Set 1   Reps: ....   (Goal: 10-20 Each Side)

Set 2   Reps: ....   (Goal: 10-20 Each Side)

Set 3   Reps: ....   (Goal: 10-20 Each Side)

Set 4   Reps: ....   (Goal: 10-20 Each Side)
(Optional)

Supersets Done Today (Circle):

1   2   3   4

 Today's Workout Intensity:

............../10

Chest & Abs

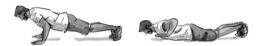

1. Stop-and-Release Push Up

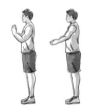

Previous Best Reps: ....
(Workout 12)

Set 1	Reps:	(Goal: 10-20)
Set 2	Reps:	(Goal: 10-20)
Set 3	Reps:	(Goal: 10-20)
Set 4	Reps:	(Goal: 10-20)
(Optional)		

2. Decline Prayers

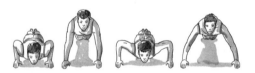

Previous Best Reps: ....
(Workout 12)

Set 1	Reps:	(Goal: 10-20)
Set 2	Reps:	(Goal: 10-20)
Set 3	Reps:	(Goal: 10-20)
Set 4	Reps:	(Goal: 10-20)
(Optional)		

3. In-And-Out Push Up

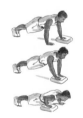

Previous Best Reps: ....
(Workout 08)

Set 1	Reps:	(Goal: 10-20)
Set 2	Reps:	(Goal: 10-20)
Set 3	Reps:	(Goal: 10-20)
Set 4	Reps:	(Goal: 10-20)
(Optional)		

4. Cross-Over-Box Push Up

Set 1	Reps:	(Goal: 10-20)
Set 2	Reps:	(Goal: 10-20)
Set 3	Reps:	(Goal: 10-20)
Set 4	Reps:	(Goal: 10-20)
(Optional)		

Make sure that you perform this exercise with controlled movements so your hands don't slip and cause injury..

5. Prayers

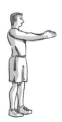

Previous Best Reps: ....
(Workout 02)

Set 1	Reps:	(Goal: 10-20)
Set 2	Reps:	(Goal: 10-20)
Set 3	Reps:	(Goal: 10-20)
Set 4	Reps:	(Goal: 10-20)
(Optional)		

  Cardio Done Today:

....

Workout 17 # Chest **& Abs**

Workout 17

Chest **& Abs**

........../........../...........
Date

1. Spider-Man Plank Crunch

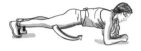
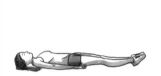

Previous Best
(Workout 14)   Reps: ....

Set 1   Reps: ....   (Goal: 10-20 Each Side)

Set 2   Reps: ....   (Goal: 10-20 Each Side)

Set 3   Reps: ....   (Goal: 10-20 Each Side)

Set 4   Reps: ....   (Goal: 10-20 Each Side)
(Optional)

2. Leg Lift

Previous Best
(Workout 14)   Reps: ....

Set 1   Reps: ....   (Goal: 10-20)

Set 2   Reps: ....   (Goal: 10-20)

Set 3   Reps: ....   (Goal: 10-20)

Set 4   Reps: ....   (Goal: 10-20)
(Optional)

3. Starfish Crunch

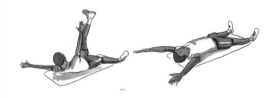

Previous Best
(Workout 09)   Reps: ....

Set 1   Reps: ....   (Goal: 10-20 Each Side)

Set 2   Reps: ....   (Goal: 10-20 Each Side)

Set 3   Reps: ....   (Goal: 10-20 Each Side)

Set 4   Reps: ....   (Goal: 10-20 Each Side)
(Optional)

4. Plank

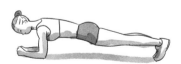

Previous Best
(Workout 14)   Reps: ....

Set 1   Time: ....   (Goal: 45-90 Seconds)

Set 2   Time: ....   (Goal: 45-90 Seconds)

Set 3   Time: ....   (Goal: 45-90 Seconds)

Set 4   Time: ....   (Goal: 45-90 Seconds)
(Optional)

 Supersets Done Today (Circle):

1   2   3   4

 89

 Today's Workout Intensity:

................/10

Back

Problem

You experience neck pain during
or after your back exercise.

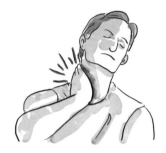

Improper form

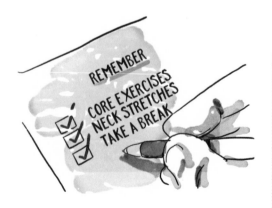

Proper form

How to Fix This

Keep your back stationary and upright –
do not move it. If you can't complete the
movement like that, go down in reps or use
an alternate exercise to strengthen your
muscles first.

Note: You may feel some of the muscles
in your upper back (specifically the
erector spinae) being worked if they're
underdeveloped as a supporting muscle.

Common Form Issue

Shoulders

Problem

You over-engage your traps, causing your shoulders to creep up to your ears.

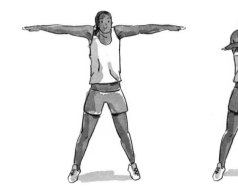

Improper form

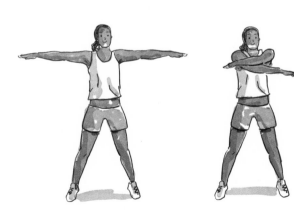

Proper form

How to Fix This

Allow your traps to fall downwards and fully disengage, isolating as much of your shoulder muscles as possible to complete the movement.

Back & Shoulders

📄 **Exercise Guide**
https://habitnest.link/WGBJ-BW18

1. Doorway Row

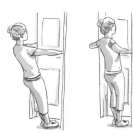

Previous Best
(Workout 11)   Reps: ....

Set 1   Reps: ....   (Goal: 10-20)

Set 2   Reps: ....   (Goal: 10-20)

Set 3   Reps: ....   (Goal: 10-20)

Set 4   Reps: ....   (Goal: 10-20)
(Optional)

2. Good Morning

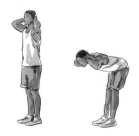

Previous Best
(Workout 06)   Reps: ....

Set 1   Reps: ....   (Goal: 10-20)

Set 2   Reps: ....   (Goal: 10-20)

Set 3   Reps: ....   (Goal: 10-20)

Set 4   Reps: ....   (Goal: 10-20)
(Optional)

3. Reverse Snow Angel

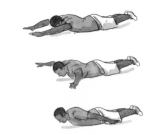

Previous Best
(Workout 06)   Reps: ....

Set 1   Reps: ....   (Goal: 10-20)

Set 2   Reps: ....   (Goal: 10-20)

Set 3   Reps: ....   (Goal: 10-20)

Set 4   Reps: ....   (Goal: 10-20)
(Optional)

4. Superman

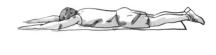
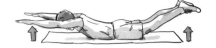

Previous Best
(Workout 11)   Reps: ....

Set 1   Reps: ....   (Goal: 10-20)

Set 2   Reps: ....   (Goal: 10-20)

Set 3   Reps: ....   (Goal: 10-20)

Set 4   Reps: ....   (Goal: 10-20)
(Optional)

🏃 Cardio Done Today:

....

Workout 18

Back **& Shoulders**

1. Side Plank + Twist

You do not want your head to go straight down in this move. Your head should go forward as you lower down.

Previous Best
(Workout 13) — Reps: ....

Set 1	Reps:	(Goal: 10-20 Each Side)
Set 2	Reps:	(Goal: 10-20 Each Side)
Set 3	Reps:	(Goal: 10-20 Each Side)
Set 4 (Optional)	Reps:	(Goal: 10-20 Each Side)

2. Y Raises

Try not to swing your arms throughout the movement.

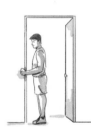

Previous Best
(Workout 13) — Reps: ....

Set 1	Reps:	(Goal: 10-20)
Set 2	Reps:	(Goal: 10-20)
Set 3	Reps:	(Goal: 10-20)
Set 4 (Optional)	Reps:	(Goal: 10-20)

3. Doorframe Hold

Previous Best
(Workout 06) — Reps: ....

Set 1	Reps:	(Goal: 10-20 Each Side)
Set 2	Reps:	(Goal: 10-20 Each Side)
Set 3	Reps:	(Goal: 10-20 Each Side)
Set 4 (Optional)	Reps:	(Goal: 10-20 Each Side)

4. Arm Scissors

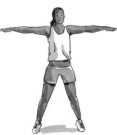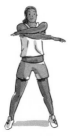

Previous Best
(Workout 04) — Reps: ....

Set 1	Reps:	(Goal: 10-20)
Set 2	Reps:	(Goal: 10-20)
Set 3	Reps:	(Goal: 10-20)
Set 4 (Optional)	Reps:	(Goal: 10-20)

Supersets Done Today (Circle):

1   2   3   4

93

 Today's Workout Intensity:

............../10

Common Form Issue

Squats

Problem

You bend your torso forward while squatting.

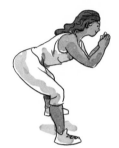
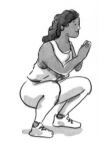

Improper form

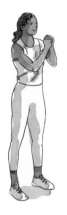
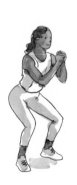

How to Fix This

Imagine a rod extending from the top of your head, down your spine, and into the floor. Engage your core as you perform your squat to help combat leaning forward, too.

Proper form

Lunges

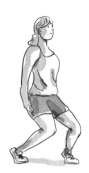

Problem

You're under-or-over-lunging. If you aren't stepping far enough, you won't get enough muscle work from the exercise. If you step too far, you will find yourself off-balance and over-extending, which can lead to injury.

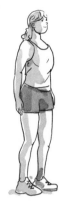

Improper form

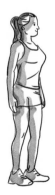

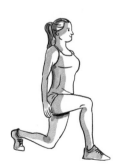

How to Fix This

The correct distance of a lunge is approximately twice your hip-width. If your heel comes off the ground, you've not stepped far enough. If your front leg shakes significantly or you need to lean, you've stepped too far.

Proper form

Legs

1. Bodyweight Deadlift

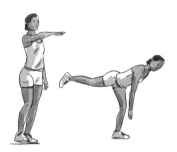

Set 1	Reps:	(Goal: 10-20 Each Side)
Set 2	Reps:	(Goal: 10-20 Each Side)
Set 3	Reps:	(Goal: 10-20 Each Side)
Set 4 (Optional)	Reps:	(Goal: 10-20 Each Side)

2. Squat

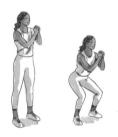

Previous Best (Workout 14)	Reps:	
Set 1	Reps:	(Goal: 10-20)
Set 2	Reps:	(Goal: 10-20)
Set 3	Reps:	(Goal: 10-20)
Set 4 (Optional)	Reps:	(Goal: 10-20)

3. Glute Bridge

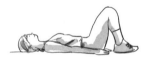
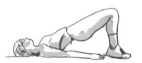

Previous Best (Workout 09)	Reps:	
Set 1	Reps:	(Goal: 10-20)
Set 2	Reps:	(Goal: 10-20)
Set 3	Reps:	(Goal: 10-20)
Set 4 (Optional)	Reps:	(Goal: 10 20)

4. Tabletop Donkey Kick

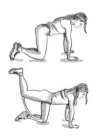

Previous Best (Workout 09)	Reps:	
Set 1	Reps:	(Goal: 10-20 Each Side)
Set 2	Reps:	(Goal: 10-20 Each Side)
Set 3	Reps:	(Goal: 10-20 Each Side)
Set 4 (Optional)	Reps:	(Goal: 10-20 Each Side)

Cardio Done Today:

....

<u>Legs</u>

5. Calf Raise

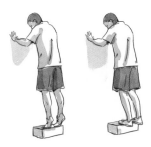

Previous Best
(Workout 14)   Reps: ....

Set 1   Reps: ....   (Goal: 10-20)

Set 2   Reps: ....   (Goal: 10-20)

Set 3   Reps: ....   (Goal: 10-20)

Set 4   Reps: ....   (Goal: 10-20)
(Optional)

6. Alternating Lunge

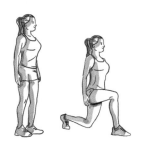

Set 1   Reps: ....   (Goal: 10-20 Each Side)

Set 2   Reps: ....   (Goal: 10-20 Each Side)

Set 3   Reps: ....   (Goal: 10-20 Each Side)

Set 4   Reps: ....   (Goal: 10-20 Each Side)
(Optional)

7. Elevated Glute Bridge

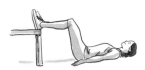

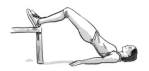

Set 1   Reps: ....   (Goal: 10-20)

Set 2   Reps: ....   (Goal: 10-20)

Set 3   Reps: ....   (Goal: 10-20)

Set 4   Reps: ....   (Goal: 10-20)
(Optional)

Supersets Done Today (Circle):

1   2   3   4

Today's Workout Intensity:

............../10

Full Body Workout

Exercise Guide
https://habitnest.link/WGBJ-BW20

Rest for **15–20 seconds between each exercise**, then rest for **1–2 minutes after completing** the entire circuit. Complete the full circuit **a total of 4–5 times**.

1. Run In Place

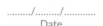

30 seconds

2. Mountain Climber

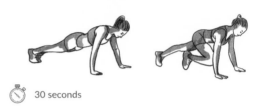

30 seconds

3. Starfish Crunch

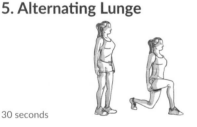

30 seconds

4. Side Plank

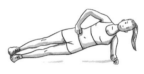

30 seconds

5. Alternating Lunge

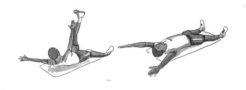

30 seconds

6. Towel Snatch

30 secon

7. Push Up

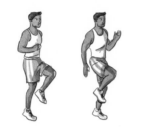

30 seconds

8. Side Plank

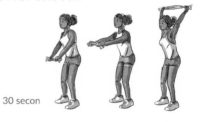

30 seconds

 Circuits Completed (Circle):

1   2   3   4   5

98

 Today's Workout Intensity:

................/10

Check-In

How am I feeling about the quality and intensity of my last 10 workouts compared to the first 10 workouts?

....

....

....

What changes am I noticing in my body?

....

....

....

When I'm working out, what takes my attention away and prevents me from being fully mentally engaged in my workouts?

....

....

....

Am I beginning to see how much I can change if I stick to this program?

....

....

....

Bonus Challenge

> *Going forward*
> *add in two supersets (four exercises)*
> *in each workout.*

This is the first optional challenge presented in this journal.

Taking this on means that in each workout, you will perform two exercises back-to-back. You'll do this twice in each workout, supersetting a total of four exercises.

Supersets work as follows: for the two exercises you're working on, you complete set one of each, back-to-back, without any rest. You rest only after finishing both, then repeat with their remaining sets. You superset 1 exercise for one muscle with 1 exercise for the other muscle being worked that day.

Supersets don't necessarily have to be done in the same order the exercises are listed on each page.

One large benefit of supersets is they **vastly** speed up your workout completion time.

Experiment with it and choose what will work best for you / your equipment.

Optional

I will complete two supersets (four exercises) each workout for the next week.

_____
↳ Signature

 Date

Back & Abs

Exercise Guide
https://habitnest.link/WGBJ-BW21

Fun Fact: Bodyweight exercises allow you to work on and perfect your form for when you perform these same exercises at the gym, with weights.

1. Simulated Pull Up

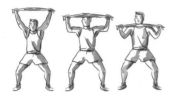

Previous Best
(Workout 11)   Reps: ....

Set 1   Reps: .... (Goal: 10-20)

Set 2   Reps: .... (Goal: 10-20)

Set 3   Reps: .... (Goal: 10-20)

Set 4   Reps: .... (Goal: 10-20)
(Optional)

2. Doorway Row

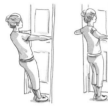

Note: You'll never fully feel ready to add challenge to an exercise. Try to challenge yourself anyway.

Previous Best
(Workout 18)   Reps: ....

Set 1   Reps: .... (Goal: 10-20)

Set 2   Reps: .... (Goal: 10-20)

Set 3   Reps: .... (Goal: 10-20)

Set 4   Reps: .... (Goal: 10-20)
(Optional)

3. Superman

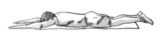
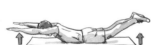

Previous Best
(Workout 18)   Reps: ....

Set 1   Reps: .... (Goal: 10-20)

Set 2   Reps: .... (Goal: 10-20)

Set 3   Reps: .... (Goal: 10-20)

Set 4   Reps: .... (Goal: 10-20)
(Optional)

4. Scapular Push Up

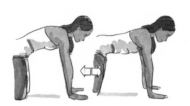

Previous Best
(Workout 11)   Reps: ....

Set 1   Reps: .... (Goal: 10-20)

Set 2   Reps: .... (Goal: 10-20)

Set 3   Reps: .... (Goal: 10-20)

Set 4   Reps: .... (Goal: 10-20)
(Optional)

5. Good Morning

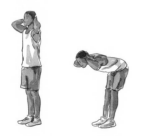

Previous Best
(Workout 18)   Reps: ....

Set 1   Reps: .... (Goal: 10-20)

Set 2   Reps: .... (Goal: 10-20)

Set 3   Reps: .... (Goal: 10-20)

Set 4   Reps: .... (Goal: 10-20)
(Optional)

Cardio Done Today:

....

Workout 21

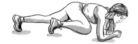

Back **& Abs**

1. Spider-Man Plank Crunch

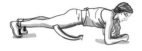

Previous Best
(Workout 17)   Reps: ....

Set 1   Reps: ....   (Goal: 10-20 Each Side)

Set 2   Reps: ....   (Goal: 10-20 Each Side)

Set 3   Reps: ....   (Goal: 10-20 Each Side)

Set 4   Reps: ....   (Goal: 10-20 Each Side)
(Optional)

2. Leg Lift

Previous Best
(Workout 17)   Reps: ....

Set 1   Reps: ....   (Goal: 10-20)

Set 2   Reps: ....   (Goal: 10-20)

Set 3   Reps: ....   (Goal: 10-20)

Set 4   Reps: ....   (Goal: 10-20)
(Optional)

3. Starfish Crunch

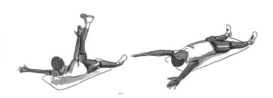

Previous Best
(Workout 17)   Reps: ....

Set 1   Reps: ....   (Goal: 10-20 Each Side)

Set 2   Reps: ....   (Goal: 10-20 Each Side)

Set 3   Reps: ....   (Goal: 10-20 Each Side)

Set 4   Reps: ....   (Goal: 10-20 Each Side)
(Optional)

4. Bicycle Crunch

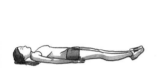

Previous Best
(Workout 14)   Reps: ....

Set 1   Reps: ....   (Goal: 10-20 Each Side)

Set 2   Reps: ....   (Goal: 10-20 Each Side)

Set 3   Reps: ....   (Goal: 10-20 Each Side)

Set 4   Reps: ....   (Goal: 10-20 Each Side)
(Optional)

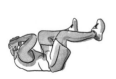 **Supersets Done Today (Circle):**

1   2   3   4

 Today's Workout Intensity:

.............../10

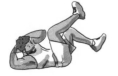

Chest & Biceps

Exercise Guide
https://habitnest.link/WGBJ-BW22

1. Stop-and-Release Push Up

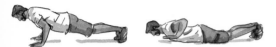

Previous Best (Workout 17)	Reps: ....
Set 1	Reps: .... (Goal: 10-20)
Set 2	Reps: .... (Goal: 10-20)
Set 3	Reps: .... (Goal: 10-20)
Set 4 (Optional)	Reps: .... (Goal: 10-20)

2. In-And-Out Push Up

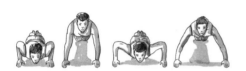

Previous Best (Workout 17)	Reps: ....
Set 1	Reps: .... (Goal: 10-20)
Set 2	Reps: .... (Goal: 10-20)
Set 3	Reps: .... (Goal: 10-20)
Set 4 (Optional)	Reps: .... (Goal: 10-20)

If you don't have an exercise ball, this can be done on the floor or a sturdy ottoman.

3. Decline Push Up

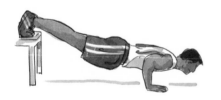

Previous Best (Workout 12)	Reps: ....
Set 1	Reps: .... (Goal: 10-20)
Set 2	Reps: .... (Goal: 10-20)
Set 3	Reps: .... (Goal: 10-20)
Set 4 (Optional)	Reps: .... (Goal: 10-20)

4. Decline Prayer

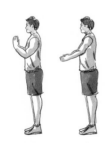

Previous Best (Workout 17)	Reps: ....
Set 1	Reps: .... (Goal: 10-20)
Set 2	Reps: .... (Goal: 10-20)
Set 3	Reps: .... (Goal: 10-20)
Set 4 (Optional)	Reps: .... (Goal: 10-20)

Cardio Done Today:

....

Workout 22

Chest **& Biceps**

1. Doorway Curl

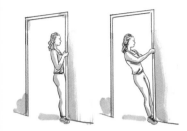

Previous Best
(Workout 12)   Reps: ....

Set 1   Reps: ....   (Goal: 10-20)

Set 2   Reps: ....   (Goal: 10-20)

Set 3   Reps: ....   (Goal: 10-20)

Set 4   Reps: ....   (Goal: 10-20)
(Optional)

2. Flexing Hammer Curl

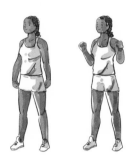

Previous Best
(Workout 16)   Reps: ....

Set 1   Reps: ....   (Goal: 10-20)

Set 2   Reps: ....   (Goal: 10-20)

Set 3   Reps: ....   (Goal: 10-20)

Set 4   Reps: ....   (Goal: 10-20)
(Optional)

3. Flexing Curl

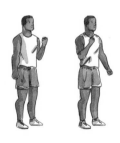

Previous Best
(Workout 16)   Reps: ....

Set 1   Reps: ....   (Goal: 10-20 Each Side)

Set 2   Reps: ....   (Goal: 10-20 Each Side)

Set 3   Reps: ....   (Goal: 10-20 Each Side)

Set 4   Reps: ....   (Goal: 10-20 Each Side)
(Optional)

4. Curl Your Leg

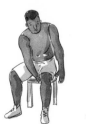
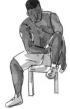

Previous Best
(Workout 16)   Reps: ....

Set 1   Reps: ....   (Goal: 10-20 Each Side)

Set 2   Reps: ....   (Goal: 10-20 Each Side)

Set 3   Reps: ....   (Goal: 10-20 Each Side)

Set 4   Reps: ....   (Goal: 10-20 Each Side)
(Optional)

Supersets Done Today (Circle):

1   2   3   4

Today's Workout Intensity:

............../10

Shoulders & Triceps

Exercise Guide
https://habitnest.link/WGBJ-BW2

1. Y Raises

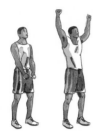

Previous Best Reps: ....
(Workout 18)

Set 1 Reps: .... (Goal: 10-20)

Set 2 Reps: .... (Goal: 10-20)

Set 3 Reps: .... (Goal: 10-20)

Set 4 Reps: .... (Goal: 10-20)
(Optional)

2. Towel Snatch

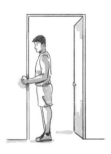

Previous Best Reps: ....
(Workout 13)

Set 1 Reps: .... (Goal: 10-20)

Set 2 Reps: .... (Goal: 10-20)

Set 3 Reps: .... (Goal: 10-20)

Set 4 Reps: .... (Goal: 10-20)
(Optional)

3. Doorframe Hold

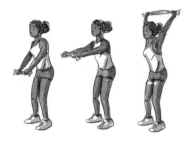

Previous Best Reps: ....
(Workout 18)

Set 1 Reps: .... (Goal: 10-20 Each Side)

Set 2 Reps: .... (Goal: 10-20 Each Side)

Set 3 Reps: .... (Goal: 10-20 Each Side)

Set 4 Reps: .... (Goal: 10-20 Each Side)
(Optional)

4. Pike Push Up

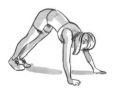
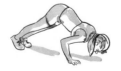

Previous Best Reps: ....
(Workout 13)

Set 1 Reps: .... (Goal: 10-20)

Set 2 Reps: .... (Goal: 10-20)

Set 3 Reps: .... (Goal: 10-20)

Set 4 Reps: .... (Goal: 10-20)
(Optional)

Cardio Done Today:

....

Workout 23   Shoulders **& Triceps**

1. Bodyweight Dips

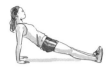
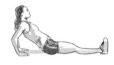

This can also be performed by resting your hands on the edge of a sturdy piece of furniture or box.

Previous Best
(Workout 16)   Reps: ....

Set 1   Reps: ....   (Goal: 10-20)

Set 2   Reps: ....   (Goal: 10-20)

Set 3   Reps: ....   (Goal: 10-20)

Set 4   Reps: ....   (Goal: 10-20)
(Optional)

2. Flexing Overhead Tricep Extension

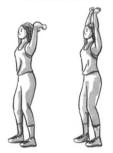

Feel free to add in descriptive notes for yourself to keep in mind, e.g. 'too easy' or 'too heavy' for the exercises. This can help you choose whether to increase reps or utilize a more challenging variation of the exercise.

Previous Best
(Workout 16)   Reps: ....

Set 1   Reps: ....   (Goal: 10-20)

Set 2   Reps: ....   (Goal: 10-20)

Set 3   Reps: ....   (Goal: 10-20)

Set 4   Reps: ....   (Goal: 10-20)
(Optional)

3. Bodyweight Skull Crusher

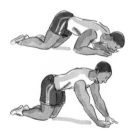

Previous Best
(Workout 16)   Reps: ....

Set 1   Reps: ....   (Goal: 10-20)

Set 2   Reps: ....   (Goal: 10-20)

Set 3   Reps: ....   (Goal: 10-20)

Set 4   Reps: ....   (Goal: 10-20)
(Optional)

4. Diamond Push Up

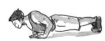

Previous Best
(Workout 16)   Reps: ....

Set 1   Reps: ....   (Goal: 10-20)

Set 2   Reps: ....   (Goal: 10-20)

Set 3   Reps: ....   (Goal: 10-20)

Set 4   Reps: ....   (Goal: 10-20)
(Optional)

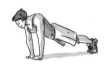 **Supersets Done Today (Circle):**

1   2   3   4

Today's Workout Intensity:

.............../10

Legs

📄 Exercise Guide
https://habitnest.link/WGBJ-BW24

1. Curtsy Lunge

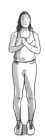
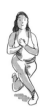

Previous Best (Workout 14)   Reps: ....

Set 1   Reps: ....   (Goal: 10-20 Each Side)

Set 2   Reps: ....   (Goal: 10-20 Each Side)

Set 3   Reps: ....   (Goal: 10-20 Each Side)

Set 4 (Optional)   Reps: ....   (Goal: 10-20 Each Side)

2. Vertical Leap

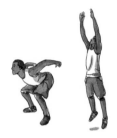

Previous Best (Workout 14)   Reps: ....

Set 1   Reps: ....   (Goal: 10-20)

Set 2   Reps: ....   (Goal: 10-20)

Set 3   Reps: ....   (Goal: 10-20)

Set 4 (Optional)   Reps: ....   (Goal: 10-20)

3. Glute Bridge

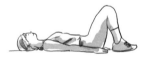
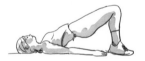

Previous Best (Workout 19)   Reps: ....

Set 1   Reps: ....   (Goal: 10-20)

Set 2   Reps: ....   (Goal: 10-20)

Set 3   Reps: ....   (Goal: 10-20)

Set 4 (Optional)   Reps: ....   (Goal: 10-20)

4. Tabletop Donkey Kick

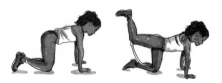

Previous Best (Workout 19)   Reps: ....

Set 1   Reps: ....   (Goal: 10-20 Each Side)

Set 2   Reps: ....   (Goal: 10-20 Each Side)

Set 3   Reps: ....   (Goal: 10-20 Each Side)

Set 4 (Optional)   Reps: ....   (Goal: 10-20 Each Side)

🏃 Cardio Done Today:

....

Legs

5. Calf Raise

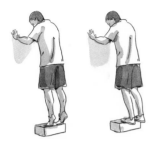

Previous Best
(Workout 19)   Reps: ....

Set 1   Reps: ....   (Goal: 10-20)

Set 2   Reps: ....   (Goal: 10-20)

Set 3   Reps: ....   (Goal: 10-20)

Set 4   Reps: ....   (Goal: 10-20)
(Optional)

6. Bodyweight Deadlift

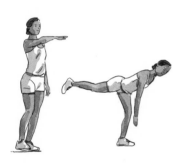

Previous Best
(Workout 19)   Reps: ....

Set 1   Reps: ....   (Goal: 10-20 Each Side)

Set 2   Reps: ....   (Goal: 10-20 Each Side)

Set 3   Reps: ....   (Goal: 10-20 Each Side)

Set 4   Reps: ....   (Goal: 10-20 Each Side)
(Optional)

7. Elevated Glute Bridge

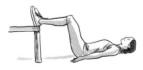
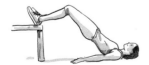

Previous Best
(Workout 19)   Reps: ....

Set 1   Reps: ....   (Goal: 10-20)

Set 2   Reps: ....   (Goal: 10-20)

Set 3   Reps: ....   (Goal: 10-20)

Set 4   Reps: ....   (Goal: 10-20)
(Optional)

Supersets Done Today (Circle):

1   2   3   4

Today's Workout Intensity:

............../10

Full Body Workout

........./........./...........
Date

Rest for **15–20 seconds between each exercise**, then rest for **1–2 minutes after completing** the entire circuit. Complete the full circuit **a total of 4–5 times**.

1. Jumping Jacks

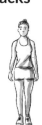
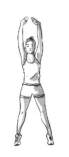

30 seconds

2. Air Squat

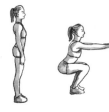

30 seconds

3. Crunch

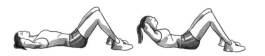

30 seconds

4. Mountain Climber

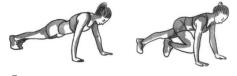

30 seconds

5. Simulated Pull Up

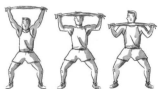
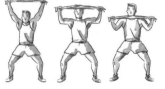

30 seconds

6. High Knee

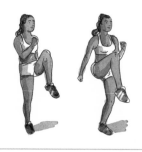

30 seconds

7. In & Out Push-Up

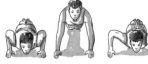
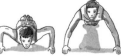
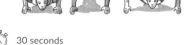

30 seconds

8. Plank

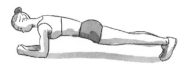

30 seconds

 Circuits Completed (Circle):

1   2   3   4   5

110

 Today's Workout Intensity:

................/10

Double Pro-Tip

> ### *Experiment with increasing your protein intake.*

Proper protein intake will make a significant, noticeable difference in your muscle growth. If you're not seeing as much muscle growth as you'd like, low protein intake could be the culprit.

As a reminder, a general standard amongst bodybuilders is to intake *0.6-0.8 (or more) grams of protein per pound of body weight.* If you are overweight, you can instead intake 1 gram per pound of lean body mass you have.

It's easy to dismiss this as being unreasonable or too hard to do, but with proper planning and food intake it becomes very doable. A large protein shake itself can provide up to 40g of protein. Adding this to your daily routine can help you hit your protein intake goals.

As always, first check with your doctor and/or a nutritionist to make sure this is appropriate for you and your body. Intaking too much protein can lead to issues, as does having protein shakes with poor-quality ingredients.

> ### *If you are overweight, make getting lean your #1 priority.*

When you are over a certain range of body fat (over 15% for males and 20% for females), your body is more likely to store excess calories as fat than as muscle.

If you fall above these ranges, you should make your first priority losing excess body fat (by being in a caloric deficit, doing consistent cardio, and doing resistance training).

Once you're leaner, you can pack on muscle much more efficiently.

Biceps & Shoulders

Exercise Guide
https://habitnest.link/WGBJ-BW26

1. Doorway Curl

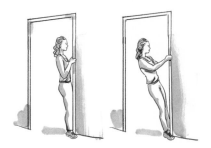

Previous Best
(Workout 22)   Reps: ....

Set 1   Reps: .... (Goal: 10-20)

Set 2   Reps: .... (Goal: 10-20)

Set 3   Reps: .... (Goal: 10-20)

Set 4   Reps: .... (Goal: 10-20)
(Optional)

2. Towel Curl

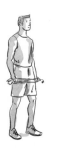
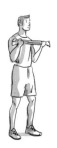

Previous Best
(Workout 16)   Reps: ....

Set 1   Reps: .... (Goal: 10-20)

Set 2   Reps: .... (Goal: 10-20)

Set 3   Reps: .... (Goal: 10-20)

Set 4   Reps: .... (Goal: 10-20)
(Optional)

*In this move, you're pulling yourself up
by the arm that's underneath your legs.*

3. Side Lying Bicep Curl

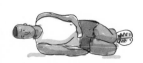
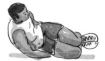

Previous Best
(Workout 07)   Reps: ....

Set 1   Reps: .... (Goal: 10-20 Each Side)

Set 2   Reps: .... (Goal: 10-20 Each Side)

Set 3   Reps: .... (Goal: 10-20 Each Side)

Set 4   Reps: .... (Goal: 10-20 Each Side)
(Optional)

4. Flexing Hammer Curl

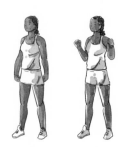

Previous Best
(Workout 22)   Reps: ....

Set 1   Reps: .... (Goal: 10-20)

Set 2   Reps: .... (Goal: 10-20)

Set 3   Reps: .... (Goal: 10-20)

Set 4   Reps: .... (Goal: 10-20)
(Optional)

Cardio Done Today:

....

Biceps **& Shoulders**

1. Y Raises

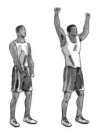

Previous Best
(Workout 23)   Reps: ....

Set 1   Reps: .... (Goal: 10-20)

Set 2   Reps: .... (Goal: 10-20)

Set 3   Reps: .... (Goal: 10-20)

Set 4   Reps: .... (Goal: 10-20)
(Optional)

2. Towel Snatch

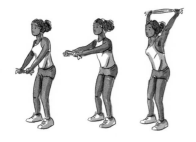

Previous Best
(Workout 23)   Reps: ....

Set 1   Reps: .... (Goal: 10-20)

Set 2   Reps: .... (Goal: 10-20)

Set 3   Reps: .... (Goal: 10-20)

Set 4   Reps: .... (Goal: 10-20)
(Optional)

3. Arm Scissors

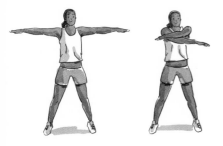

Previous Best
(Workout 18)   Reps: ....

Set 1   Reps: .... (Goal: 10-20)

Set 2   Reps: .... (Goal: 10-20)

Set 3   Reps: .... (Goal: 10-20)

Set 4   Reps: .... (Goal: 10-20)
(Optional)

4. Side Plank + Twist

Previous Best
(Workout 18)   Reps: ....

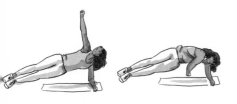

Supersets Done Today (Circle):

1   2   3   4

Today's Workout Intensity:

............../10

<u>Back</u> & Triceps

1. Simulated Pull Up

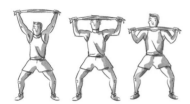

Previous Best
(Workout 21)   Reps: ....

Set 1   Reps: ....   (Goal: 10-20)

Set 2   Reps: ....   (Goal: 10-20)

Set 3   Reps: ....   (Goal: 10-20)

Set 4   Reps: ....   (Goal: 10-20)
(Optional)

2. Doorway Row

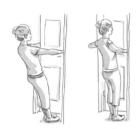

Previous Best
(Workout 21)   Reps: ....

Set 1   Reps: ....   (Goal: 10-20)

Set 2   Reps: ....   (Goal: 10-20)

Set 3   Reps: ....   (Goal: 10-20)

Set 4   Reps: ....   (Goal: 10-20)
(Optional)

3. Superman

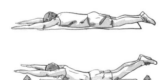

Previous Best
(Workout 21)   Reps: ....

Set 1   Reps: ....   (Goal: 10-20)

Set 2   Reps: ....   (Goal: 10-20)

Set 3   Reps: ....   (Goal: 10-20)

Set 4   Reps: ....   (Goal: 10-20)
(Optional)

4. Reverse Snow Angel

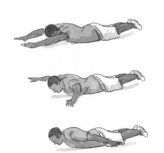

Previous Best
(Workout 18)   Reps: ....

Set 1   Reps: ....   (Goal: 10-20)

Set 2   Reps: ....   (Goal: 10-20)

Set 3   Reps: ....   (Goal: 10-20)

Set 4   Reps: ....   (Goal: 10-20)
(Optional)

Cardio Done Today:

....

Back **& Triceps**

1. Bodyweight Dips

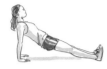

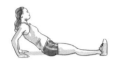

Previous Best
(Workout 23)   Reps: ....

Set 1   Reps: ....   (Goal: 10-20)

Set 2   Reps: ....   (Goal: 10-20)

Set 3   Reps: ....   (Goal: 10-20)

Set 4   Reps: ....   (Goal: 10-20)
(Optional)

2. Flexing Overhead Tricep Extension

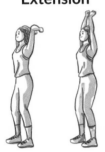

Previous Best
(Workout 23)   Reps: ....

Set 1   Reps: ....   (Goal: 10-20)

Set 2   Reps: ....   (Goal: 10-20)

Set 3   Reps: ....   (Goal: 10-20)

Set 4   Reps: ....   (Goal: 10-20)
(Optional)

3. Bodyweight Skull Crusher

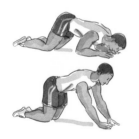

Previous Best
(Workout 23)   Reps: ....

Set 1   Reps: ....   (Goal: 10-20)

Set 2   Reps: ....   (Goal: 10-20)

Set 3   Reps: ....   (Goal: 10-20)

Set 4   Reps: ....   (Goal: 10-20)
(Optional)

4. Diamond Push Up

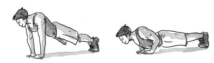

Previous Best
(Workout 23)   Reps: ....

Set 1   Reps: ....   (Goal: 10-20)

Set 2   Reps: ....   (Goal: 10-20)

Set 3   Reps: ....   (Goal: 10-20)

Set 4   Reps: ....   (Goal: 10-20)
(Optional)

Supersets Done Today (Circle):

1   2   3   4

Today's Workout Intensity:

............../10

Chest

1. Stop-and-Release Push Up

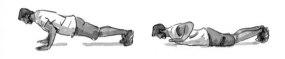

Previous Best
(Workout 22)   Reps: ....

Set 1   Reps: .... (Goal: 10-20)

Set 2   Reps: .... (Goal: 10-20)

Set 3   Reps: .... (Goal: 10-20)

Set 4   Reps: .... (Goal: 10-20)
(Optional)

2. Decline Prayers

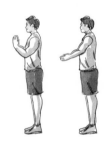

Previous Best
(Workout 17)   Reps: ....

Set 1   Reps: .... (Goal: 10-20)

Set 2   Reps: .... (Goal: 10-20)

Set 3   Reps: .... (Goal: 10-20)

Set 4   Reps: .... (Goal: 10-20)
(Optional)

*If you don't have an exercise ball, this can
be done on the floor or a sturdy ottoman.*

3. Incline Push Up

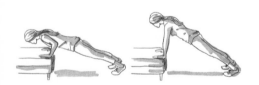

Previous Best
(Workout 12)   Reps: ....

Set 1   Reps: .... (Goal: 10-20)

Set 2   Reps: .... (Goal: 10-20)

Set 3   Reps: .... (Goal: 10-20)

Set 4   Reps: .... (Goal: 10-20)
(Optional)

4. Prayers

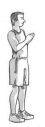 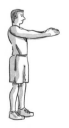

Previous Best
(Workout 17)   Reps: ....

Set 1   Reps: .... (Goal: 10-20)

Set 2   Reps: .... (Goal: 10-20)

Set 3   Reps: .... (Goal: 10-20)

Set 4   Reps: .... (Goal: 10-20)
(Optional)

🏃 Cardio Done Today:

....

Chdest

5. Push Up

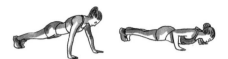

Previous Best
(Workout 08)   Reps: ....

Set 1   Reps: ....   (Goal: 10-20)

Set 2   Reps: ....   (Goal: 10-20)

Set 3   Reps: ....   (Goal: 10-20)

Set 4   Reps: ....   (Goal: 10-20)
(Optional)

6. Decline Push Up

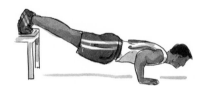

Previous Best
(Workout 22)   Reps: ....

Set 1   Reps: ....   (Goal: 10-20)

Set 2   Reps: ....   (Goal: 10-20)

Set 3   Reps: ....   (Goal: 10-20)

Set 4   Reps: ....   (Goal: 10-20)
(Optional)

7. Cross-Over-Box Push Up

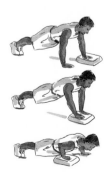

Previous Best
(Workout 17)   Reps: ....

Set 1   Reps: ....   (Goal: 10-20)

Set 2   Reps: ....   (Goal: 10-20)

Set 3   Reps: ....   (Goal: 10-20)

Set 4   Reps: ....   (Goal: 10-20)
(Optional)

Supersets Done Today (Circle):

1   2   3   4

 Today's Workout Intensity:

............../10

<u>Legs</u> & Abs

1. Bodyweight Deadlift

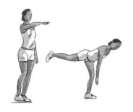

Previous Best (Workout 24)	Reps:	
Set 1	Reps:	(Goal: 10-20 Each Side)
Set 2	Reps:	(Goal: 10-20 Each Side)
Set 3	Reps:	(Goal: 10-20 Each Side)
Set 4 (Optional)	Reps:	(Goal: 10-20 Each Side)

2. Glute Bridge

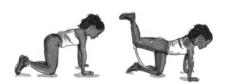

Previous Best (Workout 24)	Reps:	
Set 1	Reps:	(Goal: 10-20)
Set 2	Reps:	(Goal: 10-20)
Set 3	Reps:	(Goal: 10-20)
Set 4 (Optional)	Reps:	(Goal: 10-20)

3. Curtsy Lunge

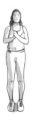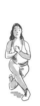

Previous Best (Workout 24)	Reps:	
Set 1	Reps:	(Goal: 10-20 Each Side)
Set 2	Reps:	(Goal: 10-20 Each Side)
Set 3	Reps:	(Goal: 10-20 Each Side)
Set 4 (Optional)	Reps:	(Goal: 10-20 Each Side)

4. Tabletop + Donkey Kick

Previous Best (Workout 24)	Reps:	
Set 1	Reps:	(Goal: 10-20 Each Side)
Set 2	Reps:	(Goal: 10-20 Each Side)
Set 3	Reps:	(Goal: 10-20 Each Side)
Set 4 (Optional)	Reps:	(Goal: 10-20 Each Side)

5. Calf Raise

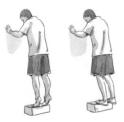

Previous Best (Workout 24)	Reps:	
Set 1	Reps:	(Goal: 10-20)
Set 2	Reps:	(Goal: 10-20)
Set 3	Reps:	(Goal: 10-20)
Set 4 (Optional)	Reps:	(Goal: 10-20)

🏃 Cardio Done Today:

....

Workout 29

Legs **& Abs**

1. Bicycle Crunch

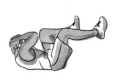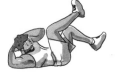

Previous Best
(Workout 21) Reps: ....

Set 1	Reps:	(Goal: 10-20 Each Side)
Set 2	Reps:	(Goal: 10-20 Each Side)
Set 3	Reps:	(Goal: 10-20 Each Side)
Set 4 (Optional)	Reps:	(Goal: 10-20 Each Side)

2. Leg Lift

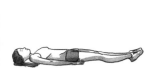

Previous Best
(Workout 21) Reps: ....

Set 1	Reps:	(Goal: 10-20)
Set 2	Reps:	(Goal: 10-20)
Set 3	Reps:	(Goal: 10-20)
Set 4 (Optional)	Reps:	(Goal: 10-20)

3. Starfish Crunch

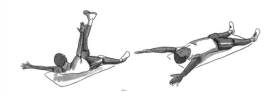

Previous Best
(Workout 21) Reps: ....

Set 1	Reps:	(Goal: 10-20 Each Side)
Set 2	Reps:	(Goal: 10-20 Each Side)
Set 3	Reps:	(Goal: 10-20 Each Side)
Set 4 (Optional)	Reps:	(Goal: 10-20 Each Side)

4. Plank

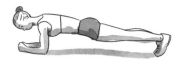

Previous Best
(Workout 17) Reps: ....

Set 1	Time:	(Goal: 45-90 Seconds)
Set 2	Time:	(Goal: 45-90 Seconds)
Set 3	Time:	(Goal: 45-90 Seconds)
Set 4 (Optional)	Time:	(Goal: 45-90 Seconds)

Supersets Done Today (Circle):

1   2   3   4

 Today's Workout Intensity:

.............../10

Full Body Workout

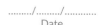
Date

Exercise Guide
https://habitnest.link/WGBJ-BW30

Rest for **15–20 seconds between each exercise**, then rest for **1–2 minutes after completing** the entire circuit. Complete the full circuit **a total of 4–5 times**.

1. Run In Place

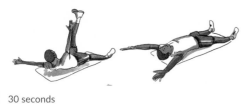

30 seconds

2. Alternating Lunge

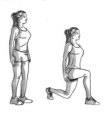

30 seconds

3. Starfish Crunch

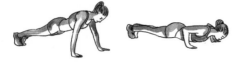

30 seconds

4. Towel Snatch

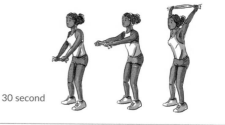

30 second

5. Push Up

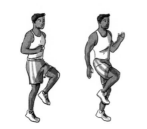

30 seconds

6. High Knee

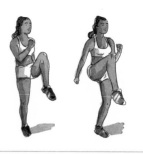

30 seconds

7. Burpee

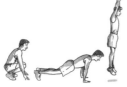

30 seconds

8. Bicycle Crunch

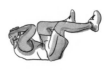
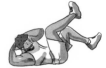

30 seconds

Circuits Completed (Circle):

1   2   3   4   5

120

Today's Workout Intensity:

................./10

Check-In

How do I feel about the way I look now compared to when I started?

....

....

....

Which body parts am I happier with?

....

....

....

Which body parts do I need to work more (maybe a bonus day for those muscles)?

....

....

....

Am I noticing any changes in my mental attitude in general (happier, more confident, etc.)?

....

....

....

Bonus Challenge

> *Going forward,*
> *complete all four sets of each exercise*
> *instead of three.*

So far in the book, we left the number of sets for each exercise as three, with the fourth being listed as optional.

This is because looking at so many sets may be overwhelming for many (8 exercises with 4 sets each = 32 sets a day!)

And it is. It's undeniably a lot of volume to pack into a workout.

But performing enough volume during workouts is one of the major keys to hypertrophy. So challenge yourself to complete four sets of four of the exercises that show up each day.

If you feel overwhelmed by this thought, consider that some of the best bodybuilders in the world perform **two full workouts a day** (yes, even those not using performance enhancing drugs).

Although that extent of exercise is a bit extreme, the results serve as a testament to the effectiveness of additional workout volume.

Optional

I will complete all four exercises of each workout from here on out.

 Signature

 Date

Chest & Abs

Exercise Guide
https://habitnest.link/WGBJ-BW31

1. Stop-and-Release Push Up

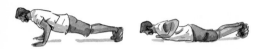

Previous Best
(Workout 28)   Reps: ....

Set 1   Reps: ....   (Goal: 10-20)

Set 2   Reps: ....   (Goal: 10-20)

Set 3   Reps: ....   (Goal: 10-20)

Set 4   Reps: ....   (Goal: 10-20)
(Optional)

2. Push Up

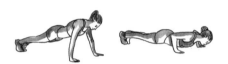

Previous Best
(Workout 28)   Reps: ....

Set 1   Reps: ....   (Goal: 10-20)

Set 2   Reps: ....   (Goal: 10-20)

Set 3   Reps: ....   (Goal: 10-20)

Set 4   Reps: ....   (Goal: 10-20)
(Optional)

3. Cross-Over-Box Push Up

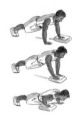

Previous Best
(Workout 28)   Reps: ....

Set 1   Reps: ....   (Goal: 10-20)

Set 2   Reps: ....   (Goal: 10-20)

Set 3   Reps: ....   (Goal: 10-20)

Set 4   Reps: ....   (Goal: 10-20)
(Optional)

4. Decline Push Up

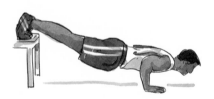

Previous Best
(Workout 28)   Reps: ....

Set 1   Reps: ....   (Goal: 10-20)

Set 2   Reps: ....   (Goal: 10-20)

Set 3   Reps: ....   (Goal: 10-20)

Set 4   Reps: ....   (Goal: 10-20)
(Optional)

5. In-And-Out Push Up

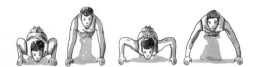

Previous Best
(Workout 22)   Reps: ....

Set 1   Reps: ....   (Goal: 10-20)

Set 2   Reps: ....   (Goal: 10-20)

Set 3   Reps: ....   (Goal: 10-20)

Set 4   Reps: ....   (Goal: 10-20)
(Optional)

Cardio Done Today:

....

Chest **& Abs**

1. Leg Lift

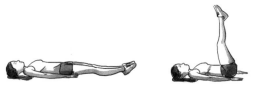

Previous Best
(Workout 29)   Reps: ....

Set 1   Reps: ....   (Goal: 10-20)

Set 2   Reps: ....   (Goal: 10-20)

Set 3   Reps: ....   (Goal: 10-20)

Set 4   Reps: ....   (Goal: 10-20)
(Optional)

2. Bicycle Crunch

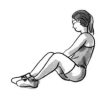 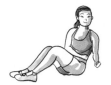

Previous Best
(Workout 29)   Reps: ....

Set 1   Reps: ....   (Goal: 10-20 Each Side)

Set 2   Reps: ....   (Goal: 10-20 Each Side)

Set 3   Reps: ....   (Goal: 10-20 Each Side)

Set 4   Reps: ....   (Goal: 10-20 Each Side)
(Optional)

3. Russian Twist

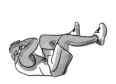 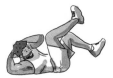

Previous Best
(Workout 11)   Reps: ....

Set 1   Reps: ....   (Goal: 10-20 Each Side)

Set 2   Reps: ....   (Goal: 10-20 Each Side)

Set 3   Reps: ....   (Goal: 10-20 Each Side)

Set 4   Reps: ....   (Goal: 10-20 Each Side)
(Optional)

4. Plank

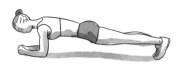

Previous Best
(Workout 29)   Time: ....

Set 1   Time: ....   (Goal: 45-90 Seconds)

Set 2   Time: ....   (Goal: 45-90 Seconds)

Set 3   Time: ....   (Goal: 45-90 Seconds)

Set 4   Time: ....   (Goal: 45-90 Seconds)
(Optional)

Supersets Done Today (Circle):

1   2   3   4

 Today's Workout Intensity:

................/10

Back & Biceps

Exercise Guide
https://habitnest.link/WGBJ-BW3

1. Simulated Pull Up

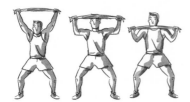

Previous Best
(Workout 27)   Reps: ....

Set 1   Reps: .... (Goal: 10-20)

Set 2   Reps: .... (Goal: 10-20)

Set 3   Reps: .... (Goal: 10-20)

Set 4   Reps: .... (Goal: 10-20)
(Optional)

2. Good Morning

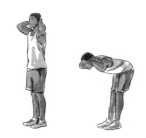

Previous Best
(Workout 21)   Reps: ....

Set 1   Reps: .... (Goal: 10-20)

Set 2   Reps: .... (Goal: 10-20)

Set 3   Reps: .... (Goal: 10-20)

Set 4   Reps: .... (Goal: 10-20)
(Optional)

3. Superman

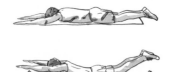

Previous Best
(Workout 27)   Reps: ....

Set 1   Reps: .... (Goal: 10-20)

Set 2   Reps: .... (Goal: 10-20)

Set 3   Reps: .... (Goal: 10-20)

Set 4   Reps: .... (Goal: 10-20)
(Optional)

4. Doorway Row

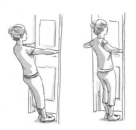

Previous Best
(Workout 27)   Reps: ....

Set 1   Reps: .... (Goal: 10-20)

Set 2   Reps: .... (Goal: 10-20)

Set 3   Reps: .... (Goal: 10-20)

Set 4   Reps: .... (Goal: 10-20)
(Optional)

Cardio Done Today:

....

Back **& Biceps**

1. Doorway Curl

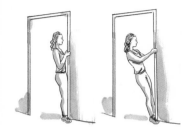

Previous Best
(Workout 26)   Reps: ....

Set 1   Reps: ....   (Goal: 10-20)

Set 2   Reps: ....   (Goal: 10-20)

Set 3   Reps: ....   (Goal: 10-20)

Set 4   Reps: ....   (Goal: 10-20)
(Optional)

2. Towel Curl

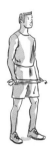
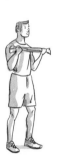

Previous Best
(Workout 26)   Reps: ....

Set 1   Reps: ....   (Goal: 10-20)

Set 2   Reps: ....   (Goal: 10-20)

Set 3   Reps: ....   (Goal: 10-20)

Set 4   Reps: ....   (Goal: 10-20)
(Optional)

3. Flexing Hammer Curl

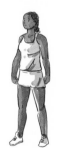
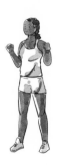

Previous Best
(Workout 26)   Reps: ....

Set 1   Reps: ....   (Goal: 10-20)

Set 2   Reps: ....   (Goal: 10-20)

Set 3   Reps: ....   (Goal: 10-20)

Set 4   Reps: ....   (Goal: 10-20)
(Optional)

4. Curl Your Leg

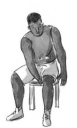
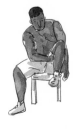

Previous Best
(Workout 22)   Reps: ....

Set 1   Reps: ....   (Goal: 10-20 Each Side)

Set 2   Reps: ....   (Goal: 10-20 Each Side)

Set 3   Reps: ....   (Goal: 10-20 Each Side)

Set 4   Reps: ....   (Goal: 10-20 Each Side)
(Optional)

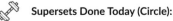

Supersets Done Today (Circle):

1   2   3   4

Today's Workout Intensity:

............../10

Shoulders & Triceps

1. Y Raises

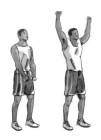

Previous Best
(Workout 26)
Reps: ....

Set 1   Reps: .... (Goal: 10-20)

Set 2   Reps: .... (Goal: 10-20)

Set 3   Reps: .... (Goal: 10-20)

Set 4   Reps: .... (Goal: 10-20)
(Optional)

2. Towel Snatch

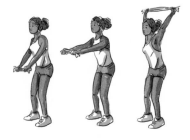

Previous Best
(Workout 26)
Reps: ....

Set 1   Reps: .... (Goal: 10-20)

Set 2   Reps: .... (Goal: 10-20)

Set 3   Reps: .... (Goal: 10-20)

Set 4   Reps: .... (Goal: 10-20)
(Optional)

3. Doorframe Hold

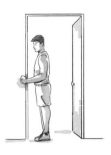

Previous Best
(Workout 23)
Reps: ....

Set 1   Reps: .... (Goal: 10-20 Each Side)

Set 2   Reps: .... (Goal: 10-20 Each Side)

Set 3   Reps: .... (Goal: 10-20 Each Side)

Set 4   Reps: .... (Goal: 10-20 Each Side)
(Optional)

4. Pike Push Up

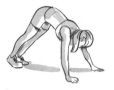
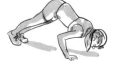

Previous Best
(Workout 23)
Reps: ....

Set 1   Reps: .... (Goal: 10-20)

Set 2   Reps: .... (Goal: 10-20)

Set 3   Reps: .... (Goal: 10-20)

Set 4   Reps: .... (Goal: 10-20)
(Optional)

Cardio Done Today:

....

Shoulders **& Triceps**

1. Bodyweight Dips

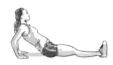

Previous Best
(Workout 27)   Reps: ....

Set 1   Reps: ....   (Goal: 10-20)

Set 2   Reps: ....   (Goal: 10-20)

Set 3   Reps: ....   (Goal: 10-20)

Set 4   Reps: ....   (Goal: 10-20)
(Optional)

2. Flexing Overhead Tricep Extension

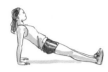

Previous Best
(Workout 27)   Reps: ....

Set 1   Reps: ....   (Goal: 10-20)

Set 2   Reps: ....   (Goal: 10-20)

Set 3   Reps: ....   (Goal: 10-20)

Set 4   Reps: ....   (Goal: 10-20)
(Optional)

3. Bodyweight Skull Crusher

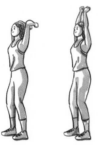

Previous Best
(Workout 27)   Reps: ....

Set 1   Reps: ....   (Goal: 10-20)

Set 2   Reps: ....   (Goal: 10-20)

Set 3   Reps: ....   (Goal: 10-20)

Set 4   Reps: ....   (Goal: 10-20)
(Optional)

4. Diamond Push Up

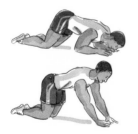

Previous Best
(Workout 27)   Reps: ....

Set 1   Reps: ....   (Goal: 10-20)

Set 2   Reps: ....   (Goal: 10-20)

Set 3   Reps: ....   (Goal: 10-20)

Set 4   Reps: ....   (Goal: 10-20)
(Optional)

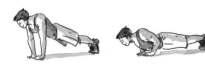

Supersets Done Today (Circle):

1   2   3   4

Today's Workout Intensity:

.............../10

Legs & Abs

1. Curtsy Lunge

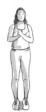
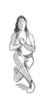

Previous Best Reps: ....
(Workout 29)

Set 1 Reps: .... (Goal: 10-20 Each Side)

Set 2 Reps: .... (Goal: 10-20 Each Side)

Set 3 Reps: .... (Goal: 10-20 Each Side)

Set 4 Reps: .... (Goal: 10-20 Each Side)
(Optional)

2. Squat

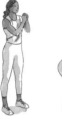
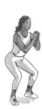

Previous Best Reps: ....
(Workout 19)

Set 1 Reps: .... (Goal: 10-20)

Set 2 Reps: .... (Goal: 10-20)

Set 3 Reps: .... (Goal: 10-20)

Set 4 Reps: .... (Goal: 10-20)
(Optional)

3. Glute Bridge

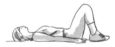
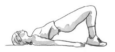

Previous Best Reps: ....
(Workout 29)

Set 1 Reps: .... (Goal: 10-20)

Set 2 Reps: .... (Goal: 10-20)

Set 3 Reps: .... (Goal: 10-20)

Set 4 Reps: .... (Goal: 10-20)
(Optional)

4. Tabletop + Donkey Kick

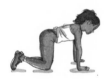
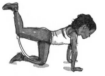

Previous Best Reps: ....
(Workout 29)

Set 1 Reps: .... (Goal: 10-20 Each Side)

Set 2 Reps: .... (Goal: 10-20 Each Side)

Set 3 Reps: .... (Goal: 10-20 Each Side)

Set 4 Reps: .... (Goal: 10-20 Each Side)
(Optional)

5. Calf Raise

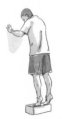
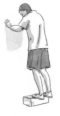

Previous Best Reps: ....
(Workout 29)

Set 1 Reps: .... (Goal: 10-20)

Set 2 Reps: .... (Goal: 10-20)

Set 3 Reps: .... (Goal: 10-20)

Set 4 Reps: .... (Goal: 10-20)
(Optional)

 Cardio Done Today:

....

Legs **& Abs**

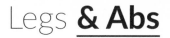

1. Spider-Man Plank Crunch

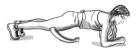
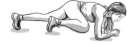

Previous Best
(Workout 21)   Reps: ....

Set 1   Reps: ....   (Goal: 10-20 Each Side)

Set 2   Reps: ....   (Goal: 10-20 Each Side)

Set 3   Reps: ....   (Goal: 10-20 Each Side)

Set 4   Reps: ....   (Goal: 10-20 Each Side)
(Optional)

2. Leg Lift

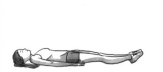

Previous Best
(Workout 31)   Reps: ....

Set 1   Reps: ....   (Goal: 10-20)

Set 2   Reps: ....   (Goal: 10-20)

Set 3   Reps: ....   (Goal: 10-20)

Set 4   Reps: ....   (Goal: 10-20)
(Optional)

3. Starfish Crunch

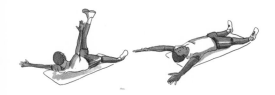

Previous Best
(Workout 29)   Reps: ....

Set 1   Reps: ....   (Goal: 10-20 Each Side)

Set 2   Reps: ....   (Goal: 10-20 Each Side)

Set 3   Reps: ....   (Goal: 10-20 Each Side)

Set 4   Reps: ....   (Goal: 10-20 Each Side)
(Optional)

4. Plank

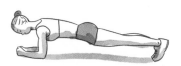

Previous Best
(Workout 31)   Reps: ....

Set 1   Time: ....   (Goal: 45-90 Seconds)

Set 2   Time: ....   (Goal: 45-90 Seconds)

Set 3   Time: ....   (Goal: 45-90 Seconds)

Set 4   Time: ....   (Goal: 45-90 Seconds)
(Optional)

Supersets Done Today (Circle):

1   2   3   4

 Today's Workout Intensity:

................/10

Full Body Workout

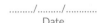
......../......../..........
Date

Rest for **15–20 seconds between each exercise**, then rest for **1–2 minutes after completing** the entire circuit. Complete the full circuit **a total of 4–5 times**.

1. Jump

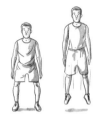

30 seconds

2. Simulated Pull Up

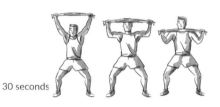

30 seconds

3. Prayers

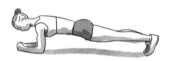

30 seconds

4. Plank

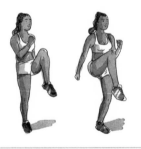

30 seconds

5. Crunch

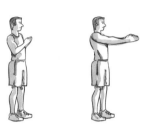

30 seconds

6. High Knee

30 seconds

7. Squat

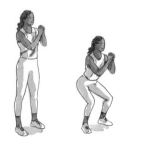

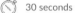
30 seconds

8. Vertical Leap

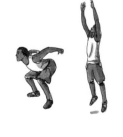

30 seconds

 Circuits Completed (Circle):

1   2   3   4   5

132

 Today's Workout Intensity:

................/10

Super Read

> ## *"Burn The Fat, Feed The Muscle"*
> ## *by Tom Venuto*

Disclaimer: We have no affiliation with Tom Venuto or his book and aren't getting paid in any way for this recommendation. It's simply a great tool.

Certain points of this journal were influenced by his book, and for good reason.

Burn The Fat, Feed The Muscle is one of the most thorough, scientifically-based books out there on fitness and nutrition.

Venuto gives all the best information out there that has been battle tested with hundreds of people and boiled down to only the most effective tips.

To take it a step further, he always creates clear, easy-to-follow action steps for most problems you'll face along this journey. He covers these for exercisers, and, particularly, lifters of all stages - beginner, intermediate, or advanced.

If you feel it would be useful for you to have a very thorough breakdown of all this, you can find his book on Amazon. It comes as a printed hardcopy, Kindle version for your phone/tablet, or audiobook.

Shoulders & Biceps

1. Y Raises

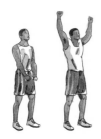

Previous Best
(Workout 33)   Reps: ....

Set 1 Reps:	(Goal: 10-20)
Set 2 Reps:	(Goal: 10-20)
Set 3 Reps:	(Goal: 10-20)
Set 4 Reps:	(Goal: 10-20)
(Optional)

2. Side Plank + Twist

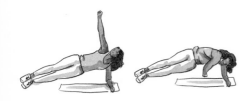

Previous Best
(Workout 26)   Reps: ....

Set 1 Reps:	(Goal: 10-20 Each Side)
Set 2 Reps:	(Goal: 10-20 Each Side)
Set 3 Reps:	(Goal: 10-20 Each Side)
Set 4 Reps:	(Goal: 10-20 Each Side)
(Optional)

3. Doorframe Hold

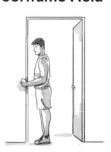

Previous Best
(Workout 33)   Reps: ....

Set 1 Reps:	(Goal: 10-20 Each Side)
Set 2 Reps:	(Goal: 10-20 Each Side)
Set 3 Reps:	(Goal: 10-20 Each Side)
Set 4 Reps:	(Goal: 10-20 Each Side)
(Optional)

4. Arm Scissors

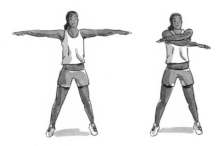

Previous Best
(Workout 26)   Reps: ....

Set 1 Reps:	(Goal: 10-20)
Set 2 Reps:	(Goal: 10-20)
Set 3 Reps:	(Goal: 10-20)
Set 4 Reps:	(Goal: 10-20)
(Optional)

Cardio Done Today:

....

Shoulders **& Biceps**

1. Doorway Curl

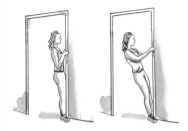

Previous Best
(Workout 32)   Reps: ....

Set 1   Reps: ....   (Goal: 10-20)

Set 2   Reps: ....   (Goal: 10-20)

Set 3   Reps: ....   (Goal: 10-20)

Set 4   Reps: ....   (Goal: 10-20)
(Optional)

2. Towel Curl

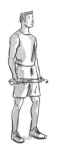
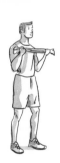

Previous Best
(Workout 32)   Reps: ....

Set 1   Reps: ....   (Goal: 10-20)

Set 2   Reps: ....   (Goal: 10-20)

Set 3   Reps: ....   (Goal: 10-20)

Set 4   Reps: ....   (Goal: 10-20)
(Optional)

3. Curl Your Leg

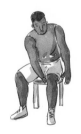
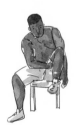

Previous Best
(Workout 32)   Reps: ....

Set 1   Reps: ....   (Goal: 10-20 Each Side)

Set 2   Reps: ....   (Goal: 10-20 Each Side)

Set 3   Reps: ....   (Goal: 10-20 Each Side)

Set 4   Reps: ....   (Goal: 10-20 Each Side)
(Optional)

4. Flexing Hammer Curl

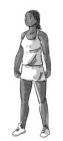
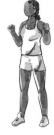
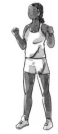

Previous Best
(Workout 32)   Reps: ....

Set 1   Reps: ....   (Goal: 10-20)

Set 2   Reps: ....   (Goal: 10-20)

Set 3   Reps: ....   (Goal: 10-20)

Set 4   Reps: ....   (Goal: 10-20)
(Optional)

Supersets Done Today (Circle):

1   2   3   4

135

 Today's Workout Intensity:

................/10

Chest & Abs

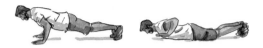

1. Stop-and-Release Push Up

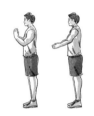

Previous Best (Workout 31)   Reps: ....

Set 1	Reps: .... (Goal: 10-20)
Set 2	Reps: .... (Goal: 10-20)
Set 3	Reps: .... (Goal: 10-20)
Set 4 (Optional)	Reps: .... (Goal: 10-20)

2. Decline Prayers

Previous Best (Workout 28)   Reps: ....

Set 1	Reps: .... (Goal: 10-20)
Set 2	Reps: .... (Goal: 10-20)
Set 3	Reps: .... (Goal: 10-20)
Set 4 (Optional)	Reps: .... (Goal: 10-20)

3. Incline Push Up

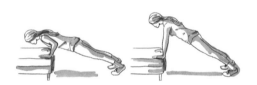

Previous Best (Workout 28)   Reps: ....

Set 1	Reps: .... (Goal: 10-20)
Set 2	Reps: .... (Goal: 10-20)
Set 3	Reps: .... (Goal: 10-20)
Set 4 (Optional)	Reps: .... (Goal: 10-20)

4. Prayers

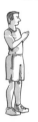
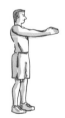

Previous Best (Workout 28)   Reps: ....

Set 1	Reps: .... (Goal: 10-20)
Set 2	Reps: .... (Goal: 10-20)
Set 3	Reps: .... (Goal: 10-20)
Set 4 (Optional)	Reps: .... (Goal: 10-20)

5. Push Up

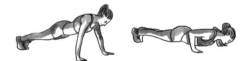

Previous Best (Workout 31)   Reps: ....

Set 1	Reps: .... (Goal: 10-20)
Set 2	Reps: .... (Goal: 10-20)
Set 3	Reps: .... (Goal: 10-20)
Set 4 (Optional)	Reps: .... (Goal: 10-20)

Cardio Done Today:

....

Chest **& Abs**

1. Spider-Man Plank Crunch

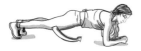
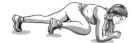

Previous Best
(Workout 34)   Reps: ....

Set 1   Reps: .... (Goal: 10-20 Each Side)

Set 2   Reps: .... (Goal: 10-20 Each Side)

Set 3   Reps: .... (Goal: 10-20 Each Side)

Set 4   Reps: .... (Goal: 10-20 Each Side)
(Optional)

2. Leg Lift

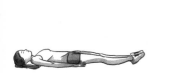

Previous Best
(Workout 34)   Reps: ....

Set 1   Reps: .... (Goal: 10-20)

Set 2   Reps: .... (Goal: 10-20)

Set 3   Reps: .... (Goal: 10-20)

Set 4   Reps: .... (Goal: 10-20)
(Optional)

3. Bicycle Crunch

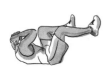
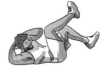

Previous Best
(Workout 34)   Reps: ....

Set 1   Reps: .... (Goal: 10-20 Each Side)

Set 2   Reps: .... (Goal: 10-20 Each Side)

Set 3   Reps: .... (Goal: 10-20 Each Side)

Set 4   Reps: .... (Goal: 10-20 Each Side)
(Optional)

4. Plank

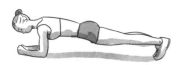

Previous Best
(Workout 34)   Reps: ....

Set 1   Time: .... (Goal: 45-90 Seconds)

Set 2   Time: .... (Goal: 45-90 Seconds)

Set 3   Time: .... (Goal: 45-90 Seconds)

Set 4   Time: .... (Goal: 45-90 Seconds)
(Optional)

Supersets Done Today (Circle):

1   2   3   4

 Today's Workout Intensity:

.............../10

Back & Triceps

Exercise Guide
https://habitnest.link/WGBJ-BW3

1. Simulated Pull Up

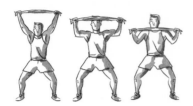

Previous Best
(Workout 32)   Reps: ....

Set 1   Reps: .... (Goal: 10-20)

Set 2   Reps: .... (Goal: 10-20)

Set 3   Reps: .... (Goal: 10-20)

Set 4   Reps: .... (Goal: 10-20)
(Optional)

2. Good Morning

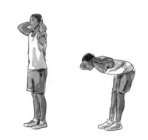

Previous Best
(Workout 32)   Reps: ....

Set 1   Reps: .... (Goal: 10-20)

Set 2   Reps: .... (Goal: 10-20)

Set 3   Reps: .... (Goal: 10-20)

Set 4   Reps: .... (Goal: 10-20)
(Optional)

3. Scapular Push Up

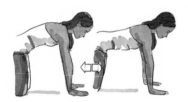

Previous Best
(Workout 21)   Reps: ....

Set 1   Reps: .... (Goal: 10-20)

Set 2   Reps: .... (Goal: 10-20)

Set 3   Reps: .... (Goal: 10-20)

Set 4   Reps: .... (Goal: 10-20)
(Optional)

4. Doorway Row

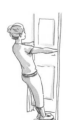
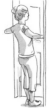

Previous Best
(Workout 32)   Reps: ....

Set 1   Reps: .... (Goal: 10-20)

Set 2   Reps: .... (Goal: 10-20)

Set 3   Reps: .... (Goal: 10-20)

Set 4   Reps: .... (Goal: 10-20)
(Optional)

Cardio Done Today:

....

Back **& Triceps**

1. Bodyweight Dips

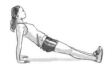

Previous Best (Workout 33)	Reps: ………………
Set 1	Reps: ……………… (Goal: 10-20)
Set 2	Reps: ……………… (Goal: 10-20)
Set 3	Reps: ……………… (Goal: 10-20)
Set 4 (Optional)	Reps: ……………… (Goal: 10-20)

2. Flexing Overhead Tricep Extension

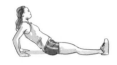

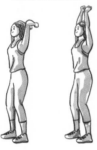

Previous Best (Workout 33)	Reps: ………………
Set 1	Reps: ……………… (Goal: 10-20)
Set 2	Reps: ……………… (Goal: 10-20)
Set 3	Reps: ……………… (Goal: 10-20)
Set 4 (Optional)	Reps: ……………… (Goal: 10-20)

3. Bodyweight Skull Crusher

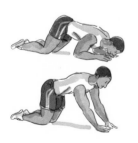

Previous Best (Workout 33)	Reps: ………………
Set 1	Reps: ……………… (Goal: 10-20)
Set 2	Reps: ……………… (Goal: 10-20)
Set 3	Reps: ……………… (Goal: 10-20)
Set 4 (Optional)	Reps: ……………… (Goal: 10-20)

4. Diamond Push Up

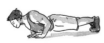

Previous Best (Workout 33)	Reps: ………………
Set 1	Reps: ……………… (Goal: 10-20)
Set 2	Reps: ……………… (Goal: 10-20)
Set 3	Reps: ……………… (Goal: 10-20)
Set 4 (Optional)	Reps: ……………… (Goal: 10-20)

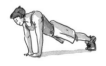 **Supersets Done Today (Circle):**

1   2   3   4

Today's Workout Intensity:

……………/10

Legs & Abs

1. Bodyweight Deadlift

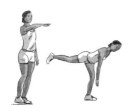

Previous Best (Workout 29)   Reps: ....

Set 1	Reps:	(Goal: 10-20 Each Side)
Set 2	Reps:	(Goal: 10-20 Each Side)
Set 3	Reps:	(Goal: 10-20 Each Side)
Set 4 (Optional)	Reps:	(Goal: 10-20 Each Side)

2. Curtsy Lunge

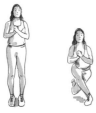

Previous Best (Workout 34)   Reps: ....

Set 1	Reps:	(Goal: 10-20 Each Side)
Set 2	Reps:	(Goal: 10-20 Each Side)
Set 3	Reps:	(Goal: 10-20 Each Side)
Set 4 (Optional)	Reps:	(Goal: 10-20 Each Side)

3. Glute Bridge

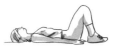
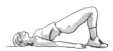

Previous Best (Workout 34)   Reps: ....

Set 1	Reps:	(Goal: 10-20)
Set 2	Reps:	(Goal: 10-20)
Set 3	Reps:	(Goal: 10-20)
Set 4 (Optional)	Reps:	(Goal: 10-20)

4. Tabletop + Donkey Kick

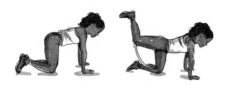

Previous Best (Workout 34)   Reps: ....

Set 1	Reps:	(Goal: 10-20 Each Side)
Set 2	Reps:	(Goal: 10-20 Each Side)
Set 3	Reps:	(Goal: 10-20 Each Side)
Set 4 (Optional)	Reps:	(Goal: 10-20 Each Side)

5. Calf Raise

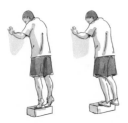

Previous Best (Workout 34)   Reps: ....

Set 1	Reps:	(Goal: 10-20)
Set 2	Reps:	(Goal: 10-20)
Set 3	Reps:	(Goal: 10-20)
Set 4 (Optional)	Reps:	(Goal: 10-20)

Cardio Done Today:

....

Legs **& Abs**

1. Spider-Man Plank Crunch

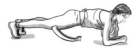

Previous Best
(Workout 37)   Reps: ....

Set 1   Reps: .... (Goal: 10-20 Each Side)

Set 2   Reps: .... (Goal: 10-20 Each Side)

Set 3   Reps: .... (Goal: 10-20 Each Side)

Set 4   Reps: .... (Goal: 10-20 Each Side)
(Optional)

2. Leg Lift

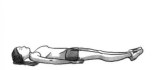

Previous Best
(Workout 37)   Reps: ....

Set 1   Reps: .... (Goal: 10-20)

Set 2   Reps: .... (Goal: 10-20)

Set 3   Reps: .... (Goal: 10-20)

Set 4   Reps: .... (Goal: 10-20)
(Optional)

3. Starfish Crunch

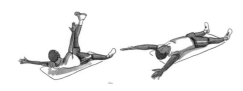

Previous Best
(Workout 34)   Reps: ....

Set 1   Reps: .... (Goal: 10-20 Each Side)

Set 2   Reps: .... (Goal: 10-20 Each Side)

Set 3   Reps: .... (Goal: 10-20 Each Side)

Set 4   Reps: .... (Goal: 10-20 Each Side)
(Optional)

4. Plank

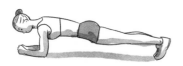

Previous Best
(Workout 37)   Reps: ....

Set 1   Time: .... (Goal: 45-90 Seconds)

Set 2   Time: .... (Goal: 45-90 Seconds)

Set 3   Time: .... (Goal: 45-90 Seconds)

Set 4   Time: .... (Goal: 45-90 Seconds)
(Optional)

Supersets Done Today (Circle):

1   2   3   4

 Today's Workout Intensity:

...............phy/10

Full Body Workout

Exercise Guide
https://habitnest.link/WGBJ-BW40

Rest for **15-20 seconds between each exercise**, then rest for **1-2 minutes after completing** the entire circuit. Complete the full circuit **a total of 4-5 times**.

1. Jumping Jack

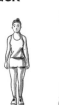

30 seconds

2. Mountain Climber

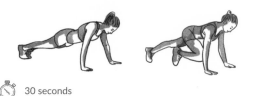

30 seconds

3. Starfish Crunch

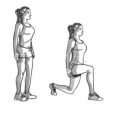

30 seconds

4. Side Plank

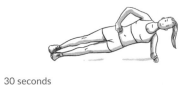

30 seconds

5. Alternating Lunge

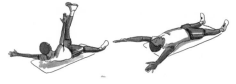

30 seconds

6. Towel Snatch

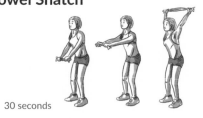

30 seconds

7. Push Up

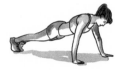

30 seconds

8. Side Plank

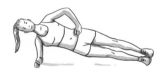

30 seconds

Circuits Completed (Circle):

142

Today's Workout Intensity:

1   2   3   4   5

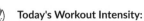

............../10

Check-In

When I'm in the middle of an exercise, am I mentally connected with the muscles that are being worked? How can I increase the quality of my mind-muscle connection during exercises?

....

....

....

Am I spending enough time focusing on the body parts I'm least satisfied with?

....

....

....

What do I love most about working out consistently?

....

....

....

How has my view of myself changed now that I've completed 40 workouts?

....

....

....

Bonus Challenge

> ### Set a long-term goal to master your eating choices one step at a time.

You already know that being on top of your nutrition goals will make a significant difference on how your body takes shape. But having perfect nutrition goes way past your body's physical manifestation.

Your daily nutrients are the source of your body's energy. The upside of mastering your nutrition is insane.

Although we built our *Nutrition Sidekick Journal* as a guide for this journey of mastery, it's not a necessity to make major shifts in your eating.

If you are not eating perfectly, there is always a reason - usually multiple. Instead of trying to change all of these eating habits at once (which is incredibly hard and impractical), we invite you to approach the process by **mastering one long-lasting change at a time.**

You may have dozens of little eating habits to change. To list some out:
- *A desire to finish everything on your plate*
- *A feeling that 'food is special / rare' and not to waste rare opportunities to eat specially-prepared food*

- *A feeling that because you ate so well during the week that you deserve to indulge more over the weekend*
- *That if your body is signaling a mood to eat something, the right move is to follow that impulse*

These are all untrue paradigms. Once you realize how to break each of them, your eyes will open to *how much happier* you can be. You will have an utter mastery of food choices and your energy.

You'll be able to walk into ANY situation, any event, and not be ruled by food, which ultimately serves YOU and your body. OWN your food, own your food choices, and you will slowly build your undeniable power over it.

Food mastery is a life-changing skill that will affect you for the rest of your life and serve as your rocket to the land of incredible physique, confidence, health, vitality, and energy.

With one change at a time, you will begin to see the momentum, impact, and level of ultimate control you have over your body and your future. Use this fuel to help feed your growth and decision making.

Optional

I will commit to being mindful of every food choice I make this week.

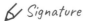 Signature

 Date

Biceps & Triceps

1. Doorway Curl

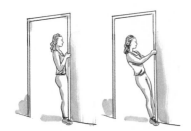

Previous Best
(Workout 36)   Reps: ....

Set 1   Reps: ....   (Goal: 10-20)

Set 2   Reps: ....   (Goal: 10-20)

Set 3   Reps: ....   (Goal: 10-20)

Set 4   Reps: ....   (Goal: 10-20)
(Optional)

2. Towel Curl

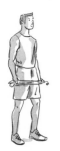
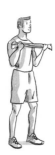

Previous Best
(Workout 36)   Reps: ....

Set 1   Reps: ....   (Goal: 10-20)

Set 2   Reps: ....   (Goal: 10-20)

Set 3   Reps: ....   (Goal: 10-20)

Set 4   Reps: ....   (Goal: 10-20)
(Optional)

3. Curl Your Leg

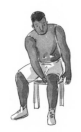
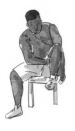

Previous Best
(Workout 36)   Reps: ....

Set 1   Reps: ....   (Goal: 10-20 Each Side)

Set 2   Reps: ....   (Goal: 10-20 Each Side)

Set 3   Reps: ....   (Goal: 10-20 Each Side)

Set 4   Reps: ....   (Goal: 10-20 Each Side)
(Optional)

4. Flexing Hammer Curl

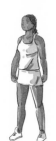
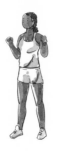

Previous Best
(Workout 36)   Reps: ....

Set 1   Reps: ....   (Goal: 10-20)

Set 2   Reps: ....   (Goal: 10-20)

Set 3   Reps: ....   (Goal: 10-20)

Set 4   Reps: ....   (Goal: 10-20)
(Optional)

Cardio Done Today:

....

Biceps **& Triceps**

1. Bodyweight Dips

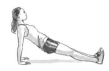
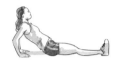

Previous Best
(Workout 38)   Reps: ....

Set 1   Reps: ....   (Goal: 10-20)

Set 2   Reps: ....   (Goal: 10-20)

Set 3   Reps: ....   (Goal: 10-20)

Set 4   Reps: ....   (Goal: 10-20)
(Optional)

2. Flexing Overhead Tricep Extension

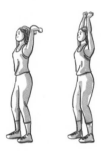

Previous Best
(Workout 38)   Reps: ....

Set 1   Reps: ....   (Goal: 10-20)

Set 2   Reps: ....   (Goal: 10-20)

Set 3   Reps: ....   (Goal: 10-20)

Set 4   Reps: ....   (Goal: 10-20)
(Optional)

3. Bodyweight Skull Crusher

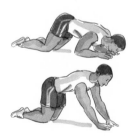

Previous Best
(Workout 38)   Reps: ....

Set 1   Reps: ....   (Goal: 10-20)

Set 2   Reps: ....   (Goal: 10-20)

Set 3   Reps: ....   (Goal: 10-20)

Set 4   Reps: ....   (Goal: 10-20)
(Optional)

4. Diamond Push Up

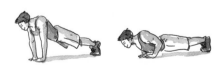

Previous Best
(Workout 38)   Reps: ....

Set 1   Reps: ....   (Goal: 10-20)

Set 2   Reps: ....   (Goal: 10-20)

Set 3   Reps: ....   (Goal: 10-20)

Set 4   Reps: ....   (Goal: 10-20)
(Optional)

Supersets Done Today (Circle):

1   2   3   4

Today's Workout Intensity:

............../10

Back & Shoulders

1. Simulated Pull Up

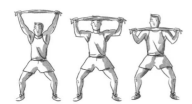

Previous Best
(Workout 38)   Reps: ....

Set 1   Reps: ....   (Goal: 10-20)

Set 2   Reps: ....   (Goal: 10-20)

Set 3   Reps: ....   (Goal: 10-20)

Set 4   Reps: ....   (Goal: 10-20)
(Optional)

2. Good Morning

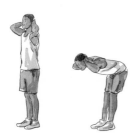

Previous Best
(Workout 38)   Reps: ....

Set 1   Reps: ....   (Goal: 10-20)

Set 2   Reps: ....   (Goal: 10-20)

Set 3   Reps: ....   (Goal: 10-20)

Set 4   Reps: ....   (Goal: 10-20)
(Optional)

3. Reverse Snow Angel

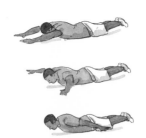

Previous Best
(Workout 27)   Reps: ....

Set 1   Reps: ....   (Goal: 10-20)

Set 2   Reps: ....   (Goal: 10-20)

Set 3   Reps: ....   (Goal: 10-20)

Set 4   Reps: ....   (Goal: 10-20)
(Optional)

4. Doorway Row

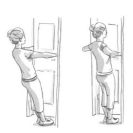

Previous Best
(Workout 38)   Reps: ....

Set 1   Reps: ....   (Goal: 10-20)

Set 2   Reps: ....   (Goal: 10-20)

Set 3   Reps: ....   (Goal: 10-20)

Set 4   Reps: ....   (Goal: 10-20)
(Optional)

Cardio Done Today:

....

Back **& Shoulders**

1. Y Raises

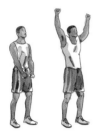

Previous Best
(Workout 36)   Reps: ....

Set 1   Reps: ....   (Goal: 10-20)

Set 2   Reps: ....   (Goal: 10-20)

Set 3   Reps: ....   (Goal: 10-20)

Set 4   Reps: ....   (Goal: 10-20)
(Optional)

2. Towel Snatch

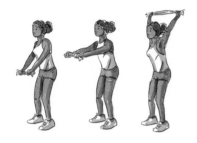

Previous Best
(Workout 33)   Reps: ....

Set 1   Reps: ....   (Goal: 10-20)

Set 2   Reps: ....   (Goal: 10-20)

Set 3   Reps: ....   (Goal: 10-20)

Set 4   Reps: ....   (Goal: 10-20)
(Optional)

3. Doorframe Hold

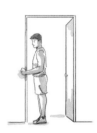

Previous Best
(Workout 36)   Reps: ....

Set 1   Reps: ....   (Goal: 10-20 Each Side)

Set 2   Reps: ....   (Goal: 10-20 Each Side)

Set 3   Reps: ....   (Goal: 10-20 Each Side)

Set 4   Reps: ....   (Goal: 10-20 Each Side)
(Optional)

4. Pike Push Up

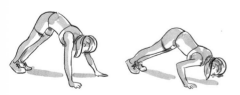

Previous Best
(Workout 33)   Reps: ....

Set 1   Reps: ....   (Goal: 10-20)

Set 2   Reps: ....   (Goal: 10-20)

Set 3   Reps: ....   (Goal: 10-20)

Set 4   Reps: ....   (Goal: 10-20)
(Optional)

Supersets Done Today (Circle):

1   2   3   4

Today's Workout Intensity:

............../10

Chest

📄 **Exercise Guide**
https://habitnest.link/WGBJ-BW43

1. Stop-and-Release Push Up

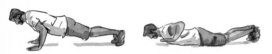

Previous Best (Workout 37)	Reps: ....
Set 1	Reps: .... (Goal: 10-20)
Set 2	Reps: .... (Goal: 10-20)
Set 3	Reps: .... (Goal: 10-20)
Set 4 (Optional)	Reps: .... (Goal: 10-20)

2. In-And-Out Push Up

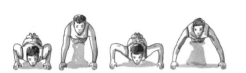

Previous Best (Workout 31)	Reps: ....
Set 1	Reps: .... (Goal: 10-20)
Set 2	Reps: .... (Goal: 10-20)
Set 3	Reps: .... (Goal: 10-20)
Set 4 (Optional)	Reps: .... (Goal: 10-20)

3. Cross-Over-Box Push Up

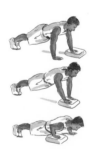

Previous Best (Workout 31)	Reps: ....
Set 1	Reps: .... (Goal: 10-20)
Set 2	Reps: .... (Goal: 10-20)
Set 3	Reps: .... (Goal: 10-20)
Set 4 (Optional)	Reps: .... (Goal: 10-20)

4. Decline Push Up

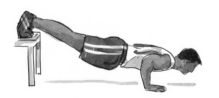

Previous Best (Workout 31)	Reps: ....
Set 1	Reps: .... (Goal: 10-20)
Set 2	Reps: .... (Goal: 10-20)
Set 3	Reps: .... (Goal: 10-20)
Set 4 (Optional)	Reps: .... (Goal: 10-20)

🏃 Cardio Done Today:

....

Chest

5. Decline Prayers

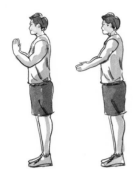

Previous Best (Workout 37)	Reps: ....
Set 1	Reps: .... (Goal: 10-20)
Set 2	Reps: .... (Goal: 10-20)
Set 3	Reps: .... (Goal: 10-20)
Set 4 (Optional)	Reps: .... (Goal: 10-20)

6. Wide-Stance Push Up

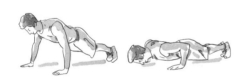

Set 1	Reps: .... (Goal: 10-20)
Set 2	Reps: .... (Goal: 10-20)
Set 3	Reps: .... (Goal: 10-20)
Set 4 (Optional)	Reps: .... (Goal: 10-20)

7. Narrow-Stance Push Up

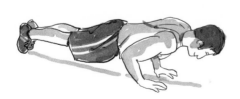

Set 1	Reps: .... (Goal: 10-20)
Set 2	Reps: .... (Goal: 10-20)
Set 3	Reps: .... (Goal: 10-20)
Set 4 (Optional)	Reps: .... (Goal: 10-20)

Supersets Done Today (Circle):

1   2   3   4

Today's Workout Intensity:

................/10

Legs & Abs

1. Bodyweight Deadlift

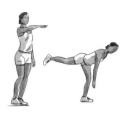

Previous Best
(Workout 39)   Reps: ....

Set 1   Reps: ....   (Goal: 10-20 Each Side)

Set 2   Reps: ....   (Goal: 10-20 Each Side)

Set 3   Reps: ....   (Goal: 10-20 Each Side)

Set 4   Reps: ....   (Goal: 10-20 Each Side)
(Optional)

2. Squat

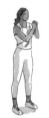
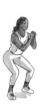

Previous Best
(Workout 34)   Reps: ....

Set 1   Reps: ....   (Goal: 10-20)

Set 2   Reps: ....   (Goal: 10-20)

Set 3   Reps: ....   (Goal: 10-20)

Set 4   Reps: ....   (Goal: 10-20)
(Optional)

3. Curtsy Lunge

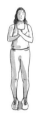
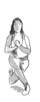

Previous Best
(Workout 39)   Reps: ....

Set 1   Reps: ....   (Goal: 10-20 Each Side)

Set 2   Reps: ....   (Goal: 10-20 Each Side)

Set 3   Reps: ....   (Goal: 10-20 Each Side)

Set 4   Reps: ....   (Goal: 10-20 Each Side)
(Optional)

4. Tabletop + Donkey Kick

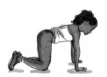
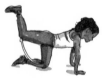

Previous Best
(Workout 39)   Reps: ....

Set 1   Reps: ....   (Goal: 10-20 Each Side)

Set 2   Reps: ....   (Goal: 10-20 Each Side)

Set 3   Reps: ....   (Goal: 10-20 Each Side)

Set 4   Reps: ....   (Goal: 10-20 Each Side)
(Optional)

5. Calf Raise

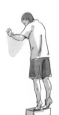
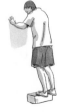

Previous Best
(Workout 39)   Reps: ....

Set 1   Reps: ....   (Goal: 10-20)

Set 2   Reps: ....   (Goal: 10-20)

Set 3   Reps: ....   (Goal: 10-20)

Set 4   Reps: ....   (Goal: 10-20)
(Optional)

Cardio Done Today:

....

Legs **& Abs**

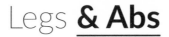

1. Spider-Man Plank Crunch

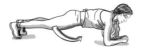
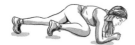

Previous Best
(Workout 39)
Reps: ……………………

Set 1   Reps: …………………   (Goal: 10-20 Each Side)

Set 2   Reps: …………………   (Goal: 10-20 Each Side)

Set 3   Reps: …………………   (Goal: 10-20 Each Side)

Set 4   Reps: …………………   (Goal: 10-20 Each Side)
(Optional)

2. Russian Twist

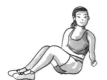

Previous Best
(Workout 31)
Reps: ……………………

Set 1   Reps: …………………   (Goal: 10-20 Each Side)

Set 2   Reps: …………………   (Goal: 10-20 Each Side)

Set 3   Reps: …………………   (Goal: 10-20 Each Side)

Set 4   Reps: …………………   (Goal: 10-20 Each Side)
(Optional)

3. Leg Lift

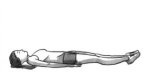

Previous Best
(Workout 39)
Reps: ……………………

Set 1   Reps: …………………   (Goal: 10-20)

Set 2   Reps: …………………   (Goal: 10-20)

Set 3   Reps: …………………   (Goal: 10-20)

Set 4   Reps: …………………   (Goal: 10-20)
(Optional)

4. Bicycle Crunch

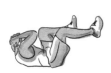
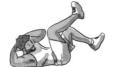

Previous Best
(Workout 37)
Reps: ……………………

Set 1   Reps: …………………   (Goal: 10-20 Each Side)

Set 2   Reps: …………………   (Goal: 10-20 Each Side)

Set 3   Reps: …………………   (Goal: 10-20 Each Side)

Set 4   Reps: …………………   (Goal: 10-20 Each Side)
(Optional)

Supersets Done Today (Circle):

1   2   3   4

 Today's Workout Intensity:

……………/10

Full Body Workout

Exercise Guide
https://habitnest.link/WGBJ-BW45

Rest for **15–20 seconds between each exercise**, then rest for **1–2 minutes after completing** the entire circuit. Complete the full circuit **a total of 4–5 times**.

1. Run In Place

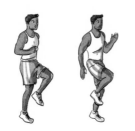

30 seconds

2. Air Squat

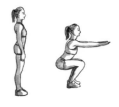

30 seconds

3. Crunch

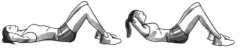

30 seconds

4. Mountain Climber

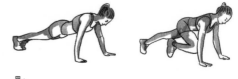

30 seconds

5. Simulated Pull Up

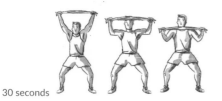

30 seconds

6. High Knee

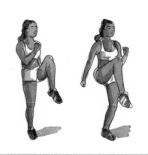

30 seconds

7. In & Out Push-Up

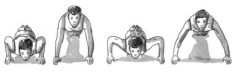

30 seconds

8. Plank

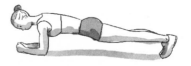

30 seconds

 Circuits Completed (Circle):   154   **Today's Workout Intensity:**

1   2   3   4   5   ..../10

Pro-Tip

> *Notice if your supporting muscles*
> *are too weak for a movement.*

If you notice you're shifting your body in weird ways and not maintaining perfect form during all points of each exercise, you are likely making this large mistake:

The body-weight you're using is enough for your main muscle (e.g. chest) **but too heavy for your underdeveloped supporting muscle** (e.g. triceps).

By knowing exactly which muscles are used in each movement, you'll be able to identify the 'weakest link' and improve the strength of that muscle by very intensely mentally focusing on its performance through each rep of your movement.

If you notice this is happening with you, an effective remedy is to add an extra day working that weak secondary muscle specifically (e.g. working triceps out 2x a week).

Alternatively, you can add 3-4 extra sets of that muscle at the end of each workout (even of different body parts) to catch it up.

To maintain form, however, consider whether or not you should implement a variation of the exercise (e.g. push ups while on knees) until you've built this muscle up.

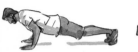 **Chest** 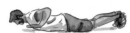 & Biceps

1. Stop-and-Release Push Up

Previous Best
(Workout 43)   Reps: ....

Set 1	Reps:	(Goal: 10-20)
Set 2	Reps:	(Goal: 10-20)
Set 3	Reps:	(Goal: 10-20)
Set 4 (Optional)	Reps:	(Goal: 10-20)

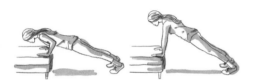

2. Incline Push Up

Previous Best
(Workout 37)   Reps: ....

Set 1	Reps:	(Goal: 10-20)
Set 2	Reps:	(Goal: 10-20)
Set 3	Reps:	(Goal: 10-20)
Set 4 (Optional)	Reps:	(Goal: 10-20)

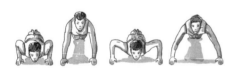

3. In-And-Out Push Up

Previous Best
(Workout 43)   Reps: ....

Set 1	Reps:	(Goal: 10-20)
Set 2	Reps:	(Goal: 10-20)
Set 3	Reps:	(Goal: 10-20)
Set 4 (Optional)	Reps:	(Goal: 10-20)

4. Prayers

Previous Best
(Workout 37)   Reps: ....

Set 1	Reps:	(Goal: 10-20)
Set 2	Reps:	(Goal: 10-20)
Set 3	Reps:	(Goal: 10-20)
Set 4 (Optional)	Reps:	(Goal: 10-20)

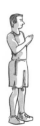 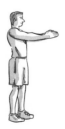

🏃 Cardio Done Today:

....

Chest **& Biceps**

1. Doorway Curl

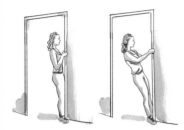

Previous Best
(Workout 41)   Reps: ....

Set 1	Reps: .... (Goal: 10-20)
Set 2	Reps: .... (Goal: 10-20)
Set 3	Reps: .... (Goal: 10-20)
Set 4
(Optional)	Reps: .... (Goal: 10-20)

2. Towel Curl

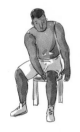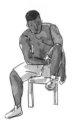

Previous Best
(Workout 41)   Reps: ....

Set 1	Reps: .... (Goal: 10-20)
Set 2	Reps: .... (Goal: 10-20)
Set 3	Reps: .... (Goal: 10-20)
Set 4
(Optional)	Reps: .... (Goal: 10-20)

3. Curl Your Leg

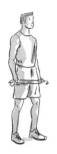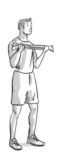

Previous Best
(Workout 41)   Reps: ....

Set 1	Reps: .... (Goal: 10-20 Each Side)
Set 2	Reps: .... (Goal: 10-20 Each Side)
Set 3	Reps: .... (Goal: 10-20 Each Side)
Set 4
(Optional)	Reps: .... (Goal: 10-20 Each Side)

4. Flexing Hammer Curl

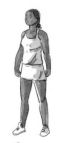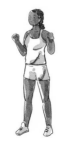

Previous Best
(Workout 41)   Reps: ....

Set 1	Reps: .... (Goal: 10-20)
Set 2	Reps: .... (Goal: 10-20)
Set 3	Reps: .... (Goal: 10-20)
Set 4
(Optional)	Reps: .... (Goal: 10-20)

Supersets Done Today (Circle):

1   2   3   4

 Today's Workout Intensity:

................/10

<u>Back</u> & Triceps

1. Doorway Row

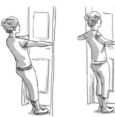

Previous Best (Workout 42)	Reps:	
Set 1	Reps:	(Goal: 10-20)
Set 2	Reps:	(Goal: 10-20)
Set 3	Reps:	(Goal: 10-20)
Set 4 (Optional)	Reps:	(Goal: 10-20)

2. Simulated Pull Up

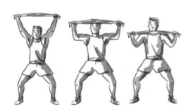

Previous Best (Workout 42)	Reps:	
Set 1	Reps:	(Goal: 10-20)
Set 2	Reps:	(Goal: 10-20)
Set 3	Reps:	(Goal: 10-20)
Set 4 (Optional)	Reps:	(Goal: 10-20)

3. Superman

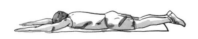
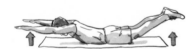

Previous Best (Workout 32)	Reps:	
Set 1	Reps:	(Goal: 10-20)
Set 2	Reps:	(Goal: 10-20)
Set 3	Reps:	(Goal: 10-20)
Set 4 (Optional)	Reps:	(Goal: 10-20)

4. Scapular Push Up

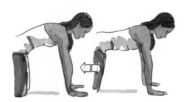

Previous Best (Workout 38)	Reps:	
Set 1	Reps:	(Goal: 10-20)
Set 2	Reps:	(Goal: 10-20)
Set 3	Reps:	(Goal: 10-20)
Set 4 (Optional)	Reps:	(Goal: 10-20)

Cardio Done Today:

....

Back **& Triceps**

1. Flexing Overhead Tricep Extension

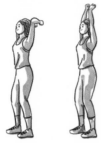

Previous Best
(Workout 41) Reps: ....

Set 1 Reps: .... (Goal: 10-20)

Set 2 Reps: .... (Goal: 10-20)

Set 3 Reps: .... (Goal: 10-20)

Set 4 Reps: .... (Goal: 10-20)
(Optional)

2. Bodyweight Dips

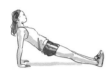
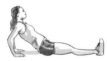

Previous Best
(Workout 41) Reps: ....

Set 1 Reps: .... (Goal: 10-20)

Set 2 Reps: .... (Goal: 10-20)

Set 3 Reps: .... (Goal: 10-20)

Set 4 Reps: .... (Goal: 10-20)
(Optional)

3. Bodyweight Skull Crusher

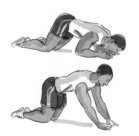

Previous Best
(Workout 41) Reps: ....

Set 1 Reps: .... (Goal: 10-20)

Set 2 Reps: .... (Goal: 10-20)

Set 3 Reps: .... (Goal: 10-20)

Set 4 Reps: .... (Goal: 10-20)
(Optional)

4. Diamond Push Up

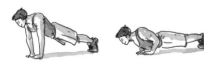

Previous Best
(Workout 41) Reps: ....

Set 1 Reps: .... (Goal: 10-20)

Set 2 Reps: .... (Goal: 10-20)

Set 3 Reps: .... (Goal: 10-20)

Set 4 Reps: .... (Goal: 10-20)
(Optional)

Supersets Done Today (Circle):

1   2   3   4

Today's Workout Intensity:

............../10

Shoulders

Exercise Guide
https://habitnest.link/WGBJ-BW48

1. Towel Snatch

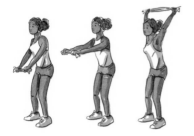

Previous Best
(Workout 42)   Reps: ....

Set 1   Reps: ....   (Goal: 10-20)

Set 2   Reps: ....   (Goal: 10-20)

Set 3   Reps: ....   (Goal: 10-20)

Set 4   Reps: ....   (Goal: 10-20)
(Optional)

2. Y Raises

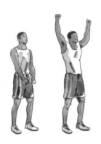

Previous Best
(Workout 42)   Reps: ....

Set 1   Reps: ....   (Goal: 10-20)

Set 2   Reps: ....   (Goal: 10-20)

Set 3   Reps: ....   (Goal: 10-20)

Set 4   Reps: ....   (Goal: 10-20)
(Optional)

3. Doorframe Hold

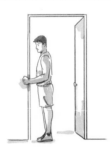

Previous Best
(Workout 42)   Reps: ....

Set 1   Reps: ....   (Goal: 10-20 Each Side)

Set 2   Reps: ....   (Goal: 10-20 Each Side)

Set 3   Reps: ....   (Goal: 10-20 Each Side)

Set 4   Reps: ....   (Goal: 10-20 Each Side)
(Optional)

4. Side Plank + Twist

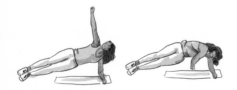

Previous Best
(Workout 36)   Reps: ....

Set 1   Reps: ....   (Goal: 10-20 Each Side)

Set 2   Reps: ....   (Goal: 10-20 Each Side)

Set 3   Reps: ....   (Goal: 10-20 Each Side)

Set 4   Reps: ....   (Goal: 10-20 Each Side)
(Optional)

Cardio Done Today:

....

Shoulders

5. Arm Scissors

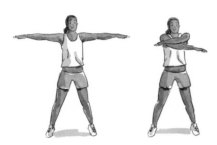

Previous Best
(Workout 36)   Reps: ....

Set 1   Reps: ....   (Goal: 10-20)

Set 2   Reps: ....   (Goal: 10-20)

Set 3   Reps: ....   (Goal: 10-20)

Set 4   Reps: ....   (Goal: 10-20)
(Optional)

6. Pike Push Up

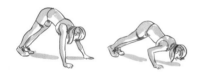

Previous Best
(Workout 42)   Reps: ....

Set 1   Reps: ....   (Goal: 10-20)

Set 2   Reps: ....   (Goal: 10-20)

Set 3   Reps: ....   (Goal: 10-20)

Set 4   Reps: ....   (Goal: 10-20)
(Optional)

7. Reverse Push Up

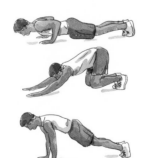

Previous Best
(Workout 04)   Reps: ....

Set 1   Reps: ....   (Goal: 10-20)

Set 2   Reps: ....   (Goal: 10-20)

Set 3   Reps: ....   (Goal: 10-20)

Set 4   Reps: ....   (Goal: 10-20)
(Optional)

Supersets Done Today (Circle):

1   2   3   4

Today's Workout Intensity:

............/10

<u>Legs</u> & Abs

1. Bodyweight Deadlift

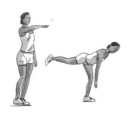

Previous Best (Workout 44)	Reps: ....
Set 1	Reps: .... (Goal: 10-20 Each Side)
Set 2	Reps: .... (Goal: 10-20 Each Side)
Set 3	Reps: .... (Goal: 10-20 Each Side)
Set 4 (Optional)	Reps: .... (Goal: 10-20 Each Side)

2. Curtsy Lunge

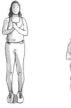

Previous Best (Workout 44)	Reps: ....
Set 1	Reps: .... (Goal: 10-20 Each Side)
Set 2	Reps: .... (Goal: 10-20 Each Side)
Set 3	Reps: .... (Goal: 10-20 Each Side)
Set 4 (Optional)	Reps: .... (Goal: 10-20 Each Side)

3. Glute Bridge

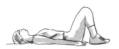

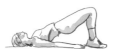

Previous Best (Workout 39)	Reps: ....
Set 1	Reps: .... (Goal: 10-20)
Set 2	Reps: .... (Goal: 10-20)
Set 3	Reps: .... (Goal: 10-20)
Set 4 (Optional)	Reps: .... (Goal: 10-20)

4. Tabletop + Donkey Kick

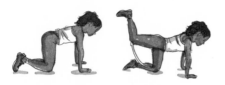

Previous Best (Workout 44)	Reps: ....
Set 1	Reps: .... (Goal: 10-20 Each Side)
Set 2	Reps: .... (Goal: 10-20 Each Side)
Set 3	Reps: .... (Goal: 10-20 Each Side)
Set 4 (Optional)	Reps: .... (Goal: 10-20 Each Side)

5. Calf Raise

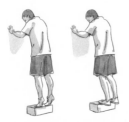

Previous Best (Workout 44)	Reps: ....
Set 1	Reps: .... (Goal: 10-20)
Set 2	Reps: .... (Goal: 10-20)
Set 3	Reps: .... (Goal: 10-20)
Set 4 (Optional)	Reps: .... (Goal: 10-20)

Cardio Done Today:

....

Legs **& Abs**

1. Spider-Man Plank Crunch

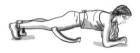

Previous Best
(Workout 44)   Reps: ....

Set 1	Reps:	(Goal: 10-20 Each Side)
Set 2	Reps:	(Goal: 10-20 Each Side)
Set 3	Reps:	(Goal: 10-20 Each Side)
Set 4 (Optional)	Reps:	(Goal: 10-20 Each Side)

2. Leg Lift

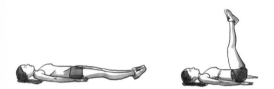

Previous Best
(Workout 44)   Reps: ....

Set 1	Reps:	(Goal: 10-20)
Set 2	Reps:	(Goal: 10-20)
Set 3	Reps:	(Goal: 10-20)
Set 4 (Optional)	Reps:	(Goal: 10-20)

3. Starfish Crunch

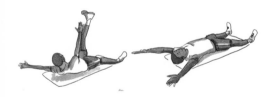

Previous Best
(Workout 39)   Reps: ....

Set 1	Reps:	(Goal: 10-20 Each Side)
Set 2	Reps:	(Goal: 10-20 Each Side)
Set 3	Reps:	(Goal: 10-20 Each Side)
Set 4 (Optional)	Reps:	(Goal: 10-20 Each Side)

4. Plank

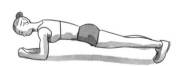

Previous Best
(Workout 39)   Reps: ....

Set 1	Time:	(Goal: 45-90 Seconds)
Set 2	Time:	(Goal: 45-90 Seconds)
Set 3	Time:	(Goal: 45-90 Seconds)
Set 4 (Optional)	Time:	(Goal: 45-90 Seconds)

Supersets Done Today (Circle):

1   2   3   4

Today's Workout Intensity:

.............../10

Full Body Workout

Exercise Guide
https://habitnest.link/WGBJ-BW50

Rest for **15-20 seconds between each exercise**, then rest for **1-2 minutes after completing** the entire circuit. Complete the full circuit **a total of 4-5 times**.

1. Jumping Jacks

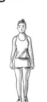
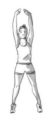

30 seconds

2. Alternating Lunge

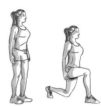

30 seconds

3. Starfish Crunch

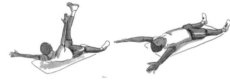
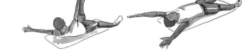

30 seconds

4. Towel Snatch

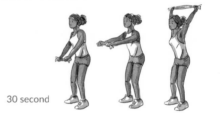

30 second

5. Push Up

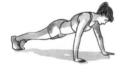
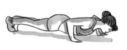

30 seconds

6. High Knee

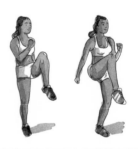

30 seconds

7. Burpee

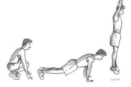

30 seconds

8. Bicycle Crunch

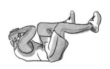
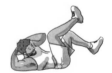

30 seconds

Circuits Completed (Circle):

1   2   3   4   5

 Today's Workout Intensity:

................/10

Check-In

How far am I from where I wanted to be when I started this journal?

....

....

....

What do I think I need to do for the next few weeks to reach my initial goal by the end of the journal?

....

....

....

Which parts of my body am I noticing significant strength gains in? Which ones are still lacking?

....

....

....

Bonus Challenge

Going forward,
complete a burn-out set, to failure,
after 4 exercises in each workout.

Burn-out sets are a fantastic way to push a muscle to a much further limit than you normally do during a workout.

This consists of doing a set normally, then very soon after, doing one more set to absolute failure.

To take your workouts to the next level, on the last, fourth set of an exercise, after a 15-20 second break, perform a burn-out set.

This only takes ~15 seconds or so each to do but will bring about an unforeseen level of intensity for that muscle as you're truly pushing it to its limit.

If you've previously taken on the other workout challenges, you can do this in addition to them. Simply choose four of the exercises each day to crush your burn-out set.

Optional

I will complete a burn-out set at the end of four different exercises during my next workout.

_____
 Signature

 Date

Back & Abs

1. Simulated Pull Up

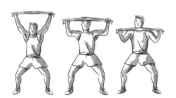

Previous Best Reps: ....
(Workout 47)

Set 1   Reps: .... (Goal: 10-20)

Set 2   Reps: .... (Goal: 10-20)

Set 3   Reps: .... (Goal: 10-20)

Set 4   Reps: .... (Goal: 10-20)
(Optional)

2. Good Morning

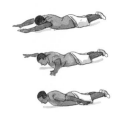

Previous Best Reps: ....
(Workout 42)

Set 1   Reps: .... (Goal: 10-20)

Set 2   Reps: .... (Goal: 10-20)

Set 3   Reps: .... (Goal: 10-20)

Set 4   Reps: .... (Goal: 10-20)
(Optional)

3. Reverse Snow Angel

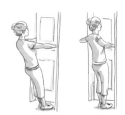

Previous Best Reps: ....
(Workout 42)

Set 1   Reps: .... (Goal: 10-20)

Set 2   Reps: .... (Goal: 10-20)

Set 3   Reps: .... (Goal: 10-20)

Set 4   Reps: .... (Goal: 10-20)
(Optional)

4. Doorway Row

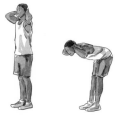

Previous Best Reps: ....
(Workout 47)

Set 1   Reps: .... (Goal: 10-20)

Set 2   Reps: .... (Goal: 10-20)

Set 3   Reps: .... (Goal: 10-20)

Set 4   Reps: .... (Goal: 10-20)
(Optional)

5. Superman

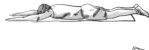

Previous Best Reps: ....
(Workout 47)

Set 1   Reps: .... (Goal: 10-20)

Set 2   Reps: .... (Goal: 10-20)

Set 3   Reps: .... (Goal: 10-20)

Set 4   Reps: .... (Goal: 10-20)
(Optional)

Cardio Done Today:

....

Back **& Abs**

1. Spider-Man Plank Crunch

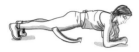
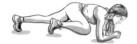

Previous Best (Workout 49)	Reps:	
Set 1	Reps:	(Goal: 10-20 Each Side)
Set 2	Reps:	(Goal: 10-20 Each Side)
Set 3	Reps:	(Goal: 10-20 Each Side)
Set 4 (Optional)	Reps:	(Goal: 10-20 Each Side)

2. Leg Lift

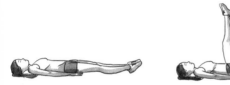

Previous Best (Workout 49)	Reps:	
Set 1	Reps:	(Goal: 10-20)
Set 2	Reps:	(Goal: 10-20)
Set 3	Reps:	(Goal: 10-20)
Set 4 (Optional)	Reps:	(Goal: 10-20)

3. Bicycle Crunch

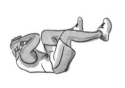
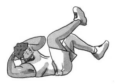

Previous Best (Workout 44)	Reps:	
Set 1	Reps:	(Goal: 10-20 Each Side)
Set 2	Reps:	(Goal: 10-20 Each Side)
Set 3	Reps:	(Goal: 10-20 Each Side)
Set 4 (Optional)	Reps:	(Goal: 10-20 Each Side)

4. Plank

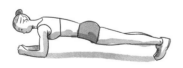

Previous Best (Workout 49)	Reps:	
Set 1	Time:	(Goal: 45-90 Seconds)
Set 2	Time:	(Goal: 45-90 Seconds)
Set 3	Time:	(Goal: 45-90 Seconds)
Set 4 (Optional)	Time:	(Goal: 45-90 Seconds)

Supersets Done Today (Circle):

1   2   3   4

Today's Workout Intensity:

................/10

<u>Chest</u> & Biceps

1. Stop-and-Release Push Up

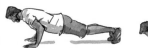
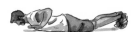

Previous Best Reps: ....
(Workout 46)

Set 1 Reps: .... (Goal: 10-20)

Set 2 Reps: .... (Goal: 10-20)

Set 3 Reps: .... (Goal: 10-20)

Set 4 Reps: .... (Goal: 10-20)
(Optional)

2. Cross-Over-Box Push Up

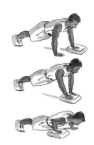

Previous Best Reps: ....
(Workout 43)

Set 1 Reps: .... (Goal: 10-20)

Set 2 Reps: .... (Goal: 10-20)

Set 3 Reps: .... (Goal: 10-20)

Set 4 Reps: .... (Goal: 10-20)
(Optional)

3. In-And-Out Push Up

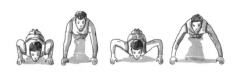

Previous Best Reps: ....
(Workout 46)

Set 1 Reps: .... (Goal: 10-20)

Set 2 Reps: .... (Goal: 10-20)

Set 3 Reps: .... (Goal: 10-20)

Set 4 Reps: .... (Goal: 10-20)
(Optional)

4. Decline Push Up

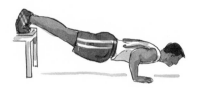

Previous Best Reps: ....
(Workout 43)

Set 1 Reps: .... (Goal: 10-20)

Set 2 Reps: .... (Goal: 10-20)

Set 3 Reps: .... (Goal: 10-20)

Set 4 Reps: .... (Goal: 10-20)
(Optional)

Cardio Done Today:

....

Chest **& Biceps**

1. Doorway Curl

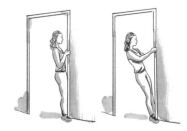

Previous Best (Workout 46) — Reps: ....

Set 1 Reps: .... (Goal: 10-20)
Set 2 Reps: .... (Goal: 10-20)
Set 3 Reps: .... (Goal: 10-20)
Set 4 (Optional) Reps: .... (Goal: 10-20)

2. Towel Curl

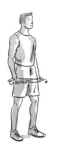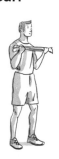

Previous Best (Workout 46) — Reps: ....

Set 1 Reps: .... (Goal: 10-20)
Set 2 Reps: .... (Goal: 10-20)
Set 3 Reps: .... (Goal: 10-20)
Set 4 (Optional) Reps: .... (Goal: 10-20)

3. Flexing Curl

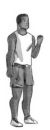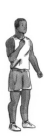

Previous Best (Workout 22) — Reps: ....

Set 1 Reps: .... (Goal: 10-20)
Set 2 Reps: .... (Goal: 10-20)
Set 3 Reps: .... (Goal: 10-20)
Set 4 (Optional) Reps: .... (Goal: 10-20)

4. Side-Lying Bicep Curl

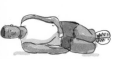

Previous Best (Workout 26) — Reps: ....

Set 1 Reps: .... (Goal: 10-20 Each Side)
Set 2 Reps: .... (Goal: 10-20 Each Side)
Set 3 Reps: .... (Goal: 10-20 Each Side)
Set 4 (Optional) Reps: .... (Goal: 10-20 Each Side)

Supersets Done Today (Circle):
1 2 3 4

Today's Workout Intensity:
............../10

Shoulders & Triceps

Exercise Guide
https://habitnest.link/WGBJ-BW5

1. Y Raises

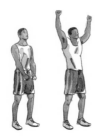

Previous Best
(Workout 48)   Reps: ....

Set 1	Reps: .... (Goal: 10-20)
Set 2	Reps: .... (Goal: 10-20)
Set 3	Reps: .... (Goal: 10-20)
Set 4 (Optional)	Reps: .... (Goal: 10-20)

2. Towel Snatch

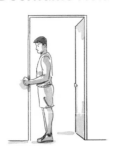

Previous Best
(Workout 48)   Reps: ....

Set 1	Reps: .... (Goal: 10-20)
Set 2	Reps: .... (Goal: 10-20)
Set 3	Reps: .... (Goal: 10-20)
Set 4 (Optional)	Reps: .... (Goal: 10-20)

3. Doorframe Hold

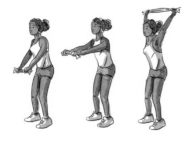

Previous Best
(Workout 48)   Reps: ....

Set 1	Reps: .... (Goal: 10-20 Each Side)
Set 2	Reps: .... (Goal: 10-20 Each Side)
Set 3	Reps: .... (Goal: 10-20 Each Side)
Set 4 (Optional)	Reps: .... (Goal: 10-20 Each Side)

4. Pike Push Up

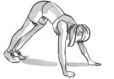
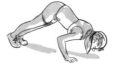

Previous Best
(Workout 48)   Reps: ....

Set 1	Reps: .... (Goal: 10-20)
Set 2	Reps: .... (Goal: 10-20)
Set 3	Reps: .... (Goal: 10-20)
Set 4 (Optional)	Reps: .... (Goal: 10-20)

Cardio Done Today:

....

Workout 53   Shoulders **& Triceps**

1. Bodyweight Dips

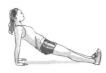
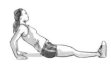

Previous Best
(Workout 47)
Reps: ....

Set 1   Reps: ....   (Goal: 10-20)

Set 2   Reps: ....   (Goal: 10-20)

Set 3   Reps: ....   (Goal: 10-20)

Set 4   Reps: ....   (Goal: 10-20)
(Optional)

2. Flexing Overhead Tricep Extension

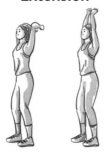

Previous Best
(Workout 47)
Reps: ....

Set 1   Reps: ....   (Goal: 10-20)

Set 2   Reps: ....   (Goal: 10-20)

Set 3   Reps: ....   (Goal: 10-20)

Set 4   Reps: ....   (Goal: 10-20)
(Optional)

3. Bodyweight Skull Crusher

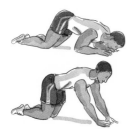

Previous Best
(Workout 47)
Reps: ....

Set 1   Reps: ....   (Goal: 10-20)

Set 2   Reps: ....   (Goal: 10-20)

Set 3   Reps: ....   (Goal: 10-20)

Set 4   Reps: ....   (Goal: 10-20)
(Optional)

4. Diamond Push Up

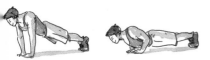

Previous Best
(Workout 47)
Reps: ....

Set 1   Reps: ....   (Goal: 10-20)

Set 2   Reps: ....   (Goal: 10-20)

Set 3   Reps: ....   (Goal: 10-20)

Set 4   Reps: ....   (Goal: 10-20)
(Optional)

Supersets Done Today (Circle):

1   2   3   4

Today's Workout Intensity:

................/10

Legs & Abs

1. Curtsy Lunge

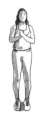
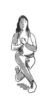

Previous Best (Workout 49)	Reps: ....
Set 1	Reps: .... (Goal: 10-20 Each Side)
Set 2	Reps: .... (Goal: 10-20 Each Side)
Set 3	Reps: .... (Goal: 10-20 Each Side)
Set 4 (Optional)	Reps: .... (Goal: 10-20 Each Side)

2. Vertical Leap

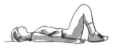

Previous Best (Workout 24)	Reps: ....
Set 1	Reps: .... (Goal: 10-20)
Set 2	Reps: .... (Goal: 10-20)
Set 3	Reps: .... (Goal: 10-20)
Set 4 (Optional)	Reps: .... (Goal: 10-20)

3. Glute Bridge

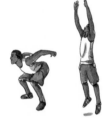
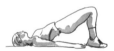

Previous Best (Workout 49)	Reps: ....
Set 1	Reps: .... (Goal: 10-20)
Set 2	Reps: .... (Goal: 10-20)
Set 3	Reps: .... (Goal: 10-20)
Set 4 (Optional)	Reps: .... (Goal: 10-20)

4. Tabletop + Donkey Kick

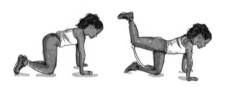

Previous Best (Workout 49)	Reps: ....
Set 1	Reps: .... (Goal: 10-20 Each Side)
Set 2	Reps: .... (Goal: 10-20 Each Side)
Set 3	Reps: .... (Goal: 10-20 Each Side)
Set 4 (Optional)	Reps: .... (Goal: 10-20 Each Side)

5. Calf Raise

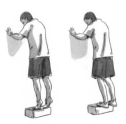

Previous Best (Workout 49)	Reps: ....
Set 1	Reps: .... (Goal: 10-20)
Set 2	Reps: .... (Goal: 10-20)
Set 3	Reps: .... (Goal: 10-20)
Set 4 (Optional)	Reps: .... (Goal: 10-20)

Cardio Done Today:

....

Legs **& Abs**

1. Spider-Man Plank Crunch

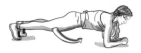
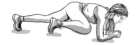

Previous Best
(Workout 51)   Reps: ....

Set 1   Reps: .... (Goal: 10-20 Each Side)

Set 2   Reps: .... (Goal: 10-20 Each Side)

Set 3   Reps: .... (Goal: 10-20 Each Side)

Set 4   Reps: .... (Goal: 10-20 Each Side)
(Optional)

2. Leg Lift

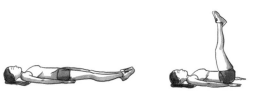

Previous Best
(Workout 51)   Reps: ....

Set 1   Reps: .... (Goal: 10-20)

Set 2   Reps: .... (Goal: 10-20)

Set 3   Reps: .... (Goal: 10-20)

Set 4   Reps: .... (Goal: 10-20)
(Optional)

3. Starfish Crunch

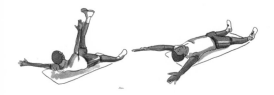

Previous Best
(Workout 49)   Reps: ....

Set 1   Reps: .... (Goal: 10-20 Each Side)

Set 2   Reps: .... (Goal: 10-20 Each Side)

Set 3   Reps: .... (Goal: 10-20 Each Side)

Set 4   Reps: .... (Goal: 10-20 Each Side)
(Optional)

4. Plank

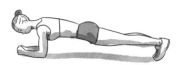

Previous Best
(Workout 51)   Reps: ....

Set 1   Time: .... (Goal: 45-90 Seconds)

Set 2   Time: .... (Goal: 45-90 Seconds)

Set 3   Time: .... (Goal: 45-90 Seconds)

Set 4   Time: .... (Goal: 45-90 Seconds)
(Optional)

Supersets Done Today (Circle):

1   2   3   4

 Today's Workout Intensity:

................/10

Full Body Workout

Exercise Guide
https://habitnest.link/WGBJ-BW55

Rest for **15-20 seconds between each exercise**, then rest for **1-2 minutes after completing** the entire circuit. Complete the full circuit **a total of 4-5 times**.

1. Jump

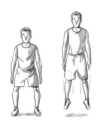

 30 seconds

2. Simulated Pull Up

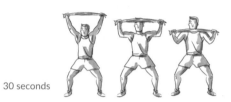

30 seconds

3. Prayers

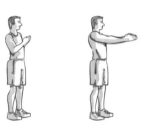

30 seconds

4. Side Plank

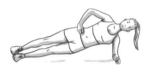

30 seconds

5. Crunch

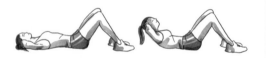

30 seconds

6. High Knee

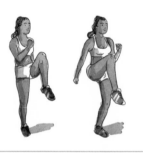

30 seconds

7. Squat

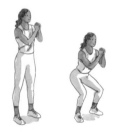

30 seconds

8. Side Plank

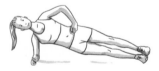

30 seconds

 Circuits Completed (Circle):

1   2   3   4   5

176

Today's Workout Intensity:

................/10

Pro-Tip

> ## *Increase your cardio if your body fat is high.*

For people trying to lose body fat - if you're at a caloric deficit, working out consistently, and still having trouble, it may be time to up your cardio.

Start by doing 20 minutes for two days a week and see how much of a difference it makes over a 1-2 week period.

If you're still not seeing visible results, up the cardio amount by one day a week, up to 6 days a week for 20 minutes each. This amount would be in addition to the body-sculpting routine listed in this journal.

If you'd like some variety from the circuit days listed in the journal, which are meant to simulate a HIIT-based cardio program

through circuit training, you can switch to running outside or using a cardio machine (ellipitical, treadmill, stair-climber, rowing machine, etc.).

You can follow a HIIT (high intensity interval training) program for any machine you choose, which shifts away from long, static cardio to bursts of intensity with recovery periods in between.

For example, one HIIT structure you could use is 30 seconds intense, 45 seconds recovery, and repeat for 20 minutes (16 cycles). Also, check out our Badass Body Goals Journal for an excellent HIIT program (https://habitnest.com).

Back & Abs

1. Simulated Pull Up

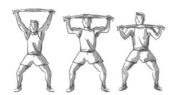

Previous Best (Workout 51)	Reps:	
Set 1	Reps:	(Goal: 10-20)
Set 2	Reps:	(Goal: 10-20)
Set 3	Reps:	(Goal: 10-20)
Set 4 (Optional)	Reps:	(Goal: 10-20)

2. Good Morning

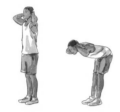

Previous Best (Workout 51)	Reps:	
Set 1	Reps:	(Goal: 10-20)
Set 2	Reps:	(Goal: 10-20)
Set 3	Reps:	(Goal: 10-20)
Set 4 (Optional)	Reps:	(Goal: 10-20)

3. Scapular Push Up

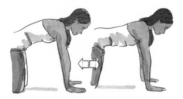

Previous Best (Workout 47)	Reps:	
Set 1	Reps:	(Goal: 10-20)
Set 2	Reps:	(Goal: 10-20)
Set 3	Reps:	(Goal: 10-20)
Set 4 (Optional)	Reps:	(Goal: 10-20)

4. Doorway Row

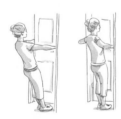

Previous Best (Workout 51)	Reps:	
Set 1	Reps:	(Goal: 10-20)
Set 2	Reps:	(Goal: 10-20)
Set 3	Reps:	(Goal: 10-20)
Set 4 (Optional)	Reps:	(Goal: 10-20)

5. Superman

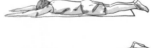

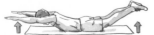

Previous Best (Workout 51)	Reps:	
Set 1	Reps:	(Goal: 10-20)
Set 2	Reps:	(Goal: 10-20)
Set 3	Reps:	(Goal: 10-20)
Set 4 (Optional)	Reps:	(Goal: 10-20)

Cardio Done Today:

....

Back **& Abs**

1. Spider-Man Plank Crunch

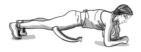

Previous Best (Workout 54)	Reps:	
Set 1	Reps:	(Goal: 10-20 Each Side)
Set 2	Reps:	(Goal: 10-20 Each Side)
Set 3	Reps:	(Goal: 10-20 Each Side)
Set 4 (Optional)	Reps:	(Goal: 10-20 Each Side)

2. Leg Lift

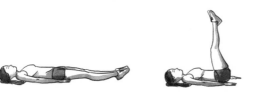

Previous Best (Workout 54)	Reps:	
Set 1	Reps:	(Goal: 10-20)
Set 2	Reps:	(Goal: 10-20)
Set 3	Reps:	(Goal: 10-20)
Set 4 (Optional)	Reps:	(Goal: 10-20)

3. Starfish Crunch

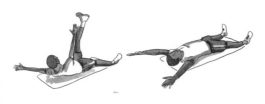

Previous Best (Workout 54)	Reps:	
Set 1	Reps:	(Goal: 10-20 Each Side)
Set 2	Reps:	(Goal: 10-20 Each Side)
Set 3	Reps:	(Goal: 10-20 Each Side)
Set 4 (Optional)	Reps:	(Goal: 10-20 Each Side)

4. Plank

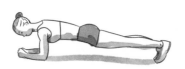

Previous Best (Workout 54)	Reps:	
Set 1	Time:	(Goal: 45-90 Seconds)
Set 2	Time:	(Goal: 45-90 Seconds)
Set 3	Time:	(Goal: 45-90 Seconds)
Set 4 (Optional)	Time:	(Goal: 45-90 Seconds)

Supersets Done Today (Circle):

1   2   3   4

Today's Workout Intensity:

............./10

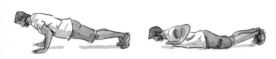

Chest & Biceps

1. Stop-and-Release Push Up

Previous Best (Workout 52)	Reps: ....
Set 1	Reps: .... (Goal: 10-20)
Set 2	Reps: .... (Goal: 10-20)
Set 3	Reps: .... (Goal: 10-20)
Set 4 (Optional)	Reps: .... (Goal: 10-20)

2. Decline Prayers

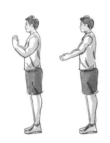

Previous Best (Workout 43)	Reps: ....
Set 1	Reps: .... (Goal: 10-20)
Set 2	Reps: .... (Goal: 10-20)
Set 3	Reps: .... (Goal: 10-20)
Set 4 (Optional)	Reps: .... (Goal: 10-20)

3. Incline Push Up

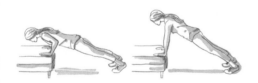

Previous Best (Workout 46)	Reps: ....
Set 1	Reps: .... (Goal: 10-20)
Set 2	Reps: .... (Goal: 10-20)
Set 3	Reps: .... (Goal: 10-20)
Set 4 (Optional)	Reps: .... (Goal: 10-20)

4. Prayers

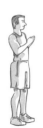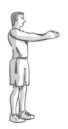

Previous Best (Workout 46)	Reps: ....
Set 1	Reps: .... (Goal: 10-20)
Set 2	Reps: .... (Goal: 10-20)
Set 3	Reps: .... (Goal: 10-20)
Set 4 (Optional)	Reps: .... (Goal: 10-20)

Cardio Done Today:

....

Chest **& Biceps**

1. Doorway Curl

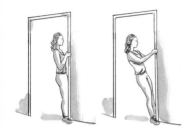

Previous Best
(Workout 52)   Reps: ....

Set 1	Reps: .... (Goal: 10-20)
Set 2	Reps: .... (Goal: 10-20)
Set 3	Reps: .... (Goal: 10-20)
Set 4 (Optional)	Reps: .... (Goal: 10-20)

2. Flexing Hammer Curl

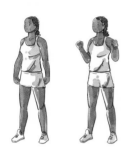

Previous Best
(Workout 46)   Reps: ....

Set 1	Reps: .... (Goal: 10-20)
Set 2	Reps: .... (Goal: 10-20)
Set 3	Reps: .... (Goal: 10-20)
Set 4 (Optional)	Reps: .... (Goal: 10-20)

3. Curl Your Leg

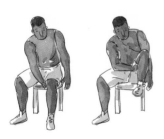

Previous Best
(Workout 46)   Reps: ....

Set 1	Reps: .... (Goal: 10-20 Each Side)
Set 2	Reps: .... (Goal: 10-20 Each Side)
Set 3	Reps: .... (Goal: 10-20 Each Side)
Set 4 (Optional)	Reps: .... (Goal: 10-20 Each Side)

4. Towel Curl

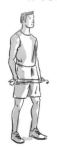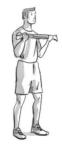

Previous Best
(Workout 52)   Reps: ....

Set 1	Reps: .... (Goal: 10-20)
Set 2	Reps: .... (Goal: 10-20)
Set 3	Reps: .... (Goal: 10-20)
Set 4 (Optional)	Reps: .... (Goal: 10-20)

Supersets Done Today (Circle):

1   2   3   4

Today's Workout Intensity:

............../10

Shoulders & Triceps

Exercise Guide
https://habitnest.link/WGBJ-BW58

1. Y Raises

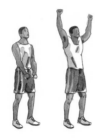

Previous Best
(Workout 53)   Reps: ....

Set 1	Reps:	(Goal: 10-20)
Set 2	Reps:	(Goal: 10-20)
Set 3	Reps:	(Goal: 10-20)
Set 4 (Optional)	Reps:	(Goal: 10-20)

2. Towel Snatch

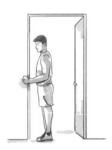

Previous Best
(Workout 53)   Reps: ....

Set 1	Reps:	(Goal: 10-20)
Set 2	Reps:	(Goal: 10-20)
Set 3	Reps:	(Goal: 10-20)
Set 4 (Optional)	Reps:	(Goal: 10-20)

3. Doorframe Hold

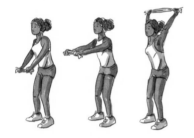

Previous Best
(Workout 53)   Reps: ....

Set 1	Reps:	(Goal: 10-20 Each Side)
Set 2	Reps:	(Goal: 10-20 Each Side)
Set 3	Reps:	(Goal: 10-20 Each Side)
Set 4 (Optional)	Reps:	(Goal: 10-20 Each Side)

4. Pike Push Up

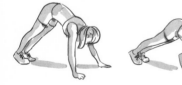

Previous Best
(Workout 53)   Reps: ....

Set 1	Reps:	(Goal: 10-20)
Set 2	Reps:	(Goal: 10-20)
Set 3	Reps:	(Goal: 10-20)
Set 4 (Optional)	Reps:	(Goal: 10-20)

Cardio Done Today:

....

Shoulders **& Triceps**

1. Bodyweight Dips

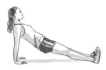

Previous Best
(Workout 53)   Reps: ....

Set 1   Reps: ....   (Goal: 10-20)

Set 2   Reps: ....   (Goal: 10-20)

Set 3   Reps: ....   (Goal: 10-20)

Set 4   Reps: ....   (Goal: 10-20)
(Optional)

2. Flexing Overhead Tricep Extension

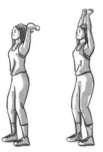

Previous Best
(Workout 53)   Reps: ....

Set 1   Reps: ....   (Goal: 10-20)

Set 2   Reps: ....   (Goal: 10-20)

Set 3   Reps: ....   (Goal: 10-20)

Set 4   Reps: ....   (Goal: 10-20)
(Optional)

3. Bodyweight Skull Crusher

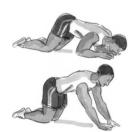

Previous Best
(Workout 53)   Reps: ....

Set 1   Reps: ....   (Goal: 10-20)

Set 2   Reps: ....   (Goal: 10-20)

Set 3   Reps: ....   (Goal: 10-20)

Set 4   Reps: ....   (Goal: 10-20)
(Optional)

4. Diamond Push Up

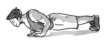

Previous Best
(Workout 53)   Reps: ....

Set 1   Reps: ....   (Goal: 10-20)

Set 2   Reps: ....   (Goal: 10-20)

Set 3   Reps: ....   (Goal: 10-20)

Set 4   Reps: ....   (Goal: 10-20)
(Optional)

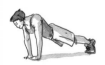 **Supersets Done Today (Circle):**

1   2   3   4

 Today's Workout Intensity:

................../10

Legs & Abs

1. Bodyweight Deadlift

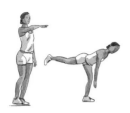

Previous Best (Workout 49)   Reps: ....

Set 1   Reps: ....   (Goal: 10-20 Each Side)

Set 2   Reps: ....   (Goal: 10-20 Each Side)

Set 3   Reps: ....   (Goal: 10-20 Each Side)

Set 4 (Optional)   Reps: ....   (Goal: 10-20 Each Side)

2. Glute Bridge

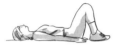
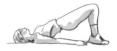

Previous Best (Workout 54)   Reps: ....

Set 1   Reps: ....   (Goal: 10-20)

Set 2   Reps: ....   (Goal: 10-20)

Set 3   Reps: ....   (Goal: 10-20)

Set 4 (Optional)   Reps: ....   (Goal: 10-20)

3. Curtsy Lunge

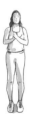
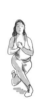

Previous Best (Workout 54)   Reps: ....

Set 1   Reps: ....   (Goal: 10-20 Each Side)

Set 2   Reps: ....   (Goal: 10-20 Each Side)

Set 3   Reps: ....   (Goal: 10-20 Each Side)

Set 4 (Optional)   Reps: ....   (Goal: 10-20 Each Side)

4. Tabletop + Donkey Kick

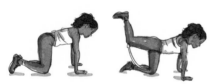

Previous Best (Workout 54)   Reps: ....

Set 1   Reps: ....   (Goal: 10-20 Each Side)

Set 2   Reps: ....   (Goal: 10-20 Each Side)

Set 3   Reps: ....   (Goal: 10-20 Each Side)

Set 4 (Optional)   Reps: ....   (Goal: 10-20 Each Side)

5. Calf Raise

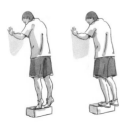

Previous Best (Workout 54)   Reps: ....

Set 1   Reps: ....   (Goal: 10-20)

Set 2   Reps: ....   (Goal: 10-20)

Set 3   Reps: ....   (Goal: 10-20)

Set 4 (Optional)   Reps: ....   (Goal: 10-20)

Cardio Done Today:

....

Legs **& Abs**

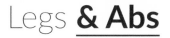

........../.........../............
Date

1. Spider-Man Plank Crunch

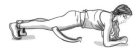

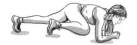

Previous Best
(Workout 56)   Reps: ....

Set 1   Reps: ....   (Goal: 10-20 Each Side)

Set 2   Reps: ....   (Goal: 10-20 Each Side)

Set 3   Reps: ....   (Goal: 10-20 Each Side)

Set 4   Reps: ....   (Goal: 10-20 Each Side)
(Optional)

2. Leg Lift

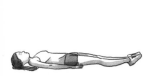

Previous Best
(Workout 56)   Reps: ....

Set 1   Reps: ....   (Goal: 10-20)

Set 2   Reps: ....   (Goal: 10-20)

Set 3   Reps: ....   (Goal: 10-20)

Set 4   Reps: ....   (Goal: 10-20)
(Optional)

3. Bicycle Crunch

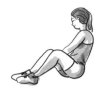
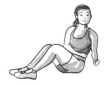

Previous Best
(Workout 44)   Reps: ....

Set 1   Reps: ....   (Goal: 10-20 Each Side)

Set 2   Reps: ....   (Goal: 10-20 Each Side)

Set 3   Reps: ....   (Goal: 10-20 Each Side)

Set 4   Reps: ....   (Goal: 10-20 Each Side)
(Optional)

4. Plank

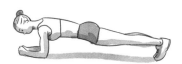

Previous Best
(Workout 56)   Reps: ....

Set 1   Time: ....   (Goal: 45-90 Seconds)

Set 2   Time: ....   (Goal: 45-90 Seconds)

Set 3   Time: ....   (Goal: 45-90 Seconds)

Set 4   Time: ....   (Goal: 45-90 Seconds)
(Optional)

Supersets Done Today (Circle):

1   2   3   4

 Today's Workout Intensity:

................./10

Full Body Workout

Exercise Guide
https://habitnest.link/WGBJ-BW60

Rest for **15-20 seconds between each exercise**, then rest for **1-2 minutes after completing** the entire circuit. Complete the full circuit **a total of 4-5 times**.

1. Run In Place

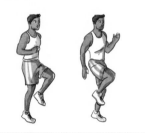

⏱ 30 seconds

2. Mountain Climber

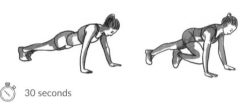

⏱ 30 seconds

3. Starfish Crunch

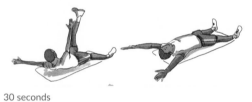

⏱ 30 seconds

4. Bicycle Crunch

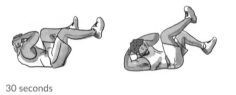

⏱ 30 seconds

5. Alternating Lunge

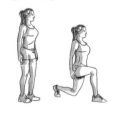

⏱ 30 seconds

6. Towel Snatch

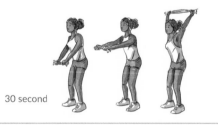

⏱ 30 second

7. Push Up

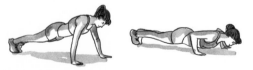

⏱ 30 seconds

8. Vertical Leap

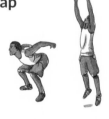

⏱ 30 seconds

↻ **Circuits Completed (Circle):**

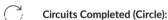
1   2   3   4   5

 Today's Workout Intensity:

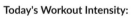
............../10

Check-In

How do I feel about the way I look now compared to when I started?

....

....

....

Which body parts am I happier with?

....

....

....

Which body parts do I need to work more (maybe a bonus day for those muscles)?

....

....

....

Am I noticing any changes in my mental attitude in general (happier, more confident, etc.)?

....

....

....

Back & Abs

1. Simulated Pull Up

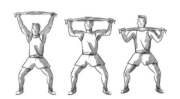

Previous Best
(Workout 56)   Reps: ....

Set 1	Reps:	(Goal: 10-20)
Set 2	Reps:	(Goal: 10-20)
Set 3	Reps:	(Goal: 10-20)
Set 4
(Optional)	Reps:	(Goal: 10-20)

2. Good Morning

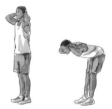

Previous Best
(Workout 56)   Reps: ....

Set 1	Reps:	(Goal: 10-20)
Set 2	Reps:	(Goal: 10-20)
Set 3	Reps:	(Goal: 10-20)
Set 4
(Optional)	Reps:	(Goal: 10-20)

3. Reverse Snow Angel

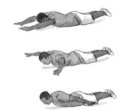

Previous Best
(Workout 51)   Reps: ....

Set 1	Reps:	(Goal: 10-20)
Set 2	Reps:	(Goal: 10-20)
Set 3	Reps:	(Goal: 10-20)
Set 4
(Optional)	Reps:	(Goal: 10-20)

4. Doorway Row

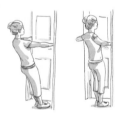

Previous Best
(Workout 56)   Reps: ....

Set 1	Reps:	(Goal: 10-20)
Set 2	Reps:	(Goal: 10-20)
Set 3	Reps:	(Goal: 10-20)
Set 4
(Optional)	Reps:	(Goal: 10-20)

5. Superman

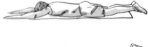

Previous Best
(Workout 56)   Reps: ....

Set 1	Reps:	(Goal: 10-20)
Set 2	Reps:	(Goal: 10-20)
Set 3	Reps:	(Goal: 10-20)
Set 4
(Optional)	Reps:	(Goal: 10-20)

Cardio Done Today:
....

Back **& Abs**

1. Spider-Man Plank Crunch

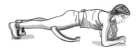
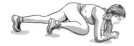

Previous Best
(Workout 59)
Reps: ....

Set 1	Reps:	(Goal: 10-20 Each Side)
Set 2	Reps:	(Goal: 10-20 Each Side)
Set 3	Reps:	(Goal: 10-20 Each Side)
Set 4 (Optional)	Reps:	(Goal: 10-20 Each Side)

2. Leg Lift

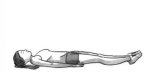

Previous Best
(Workout 59)
Reps: ....

Set 1	Reps:	(Goal: 10-20)
Set 2	Reps:	(Goal: 10-20)
Set 3	Reps:	(Goal: 10-20)
Set 4 (Optional)	Reps:	(Goal: 10-20)

3. Starfish Crunch

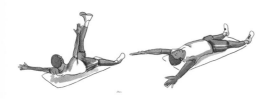

Previous Best
(Workout 56)
Reps: ....

Set 1	Reps:	(Goal: 10-20 Each Side)
Set 2	Reps:	(Goal: 10-20 Each Side)
Set 3	Reps:	(Goal: 10-20 Each Side)
Set 4 (Optional)	Reps:	(Goal: 10-20 Each Side)

4. Plank

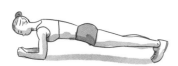

Previous Best
(Workout 59)
Reps: ....

Set 1	Time:	(Goal: 45-90 Seconds)
Set 2	Time:	(Goal: 45-90 Seconds)
Set 3	Time:	(Goal: 45-90 Seconds)
Set 4 (Optional)	Time:	(Goal: 45-90 Seconds)

Supersets Done Today (Circle):

1   2   3   4

Today's Workout Intensity:

................/10

Chest & Biceps

1. Stop-and-Release Push Up

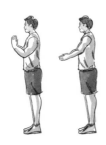

Previous Best
(Workout 57)   Reps: ....

Set 1   Reps: ....   (Goal: 10-20)

Set 2   Reps: ....   (Goal: 10-20)

Set 3   Reps: ....   (Goal: 10-20)

Set 4   Reps: ....   (Goal: 10-20)
(Optional)

2. Decline Prayers

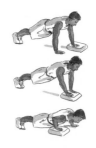

Previous Best
(Workout 57)   Reps: ....

Set 1   Reps: ....   (Goal: 10-20)

Set 2   Reps: ....   (Goal: 10-20)

Set 3   Reps: ....   (Goal: 10-20)

Set 4   Reps: ....   (Goal: 10-20)
(Optional)

3. Cross-Over-Box Push Up

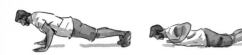

Previous Best
(Workout 52)   Reps: ....

Set 1   Reps: ....   (Goal: 10-20)

Set 2   Reps: ....   (Goal: 10-20)

Set 3   Reps: ....   (Goal: 10-20)

Set 4   Reps: ....   (Goal: 10-20)
(Optional)

4. Decline Push Up

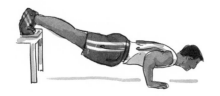

Previous Best
(Workout 57)   Reps: ....

Set 1   Reps: ....   (Goal: 10-20)

Set 2   Reps: ....   (Goal: 10-20)

Set 3   Reps: ....   (Goal: 10-20)

Set 4   Reps: ....   (Goal: 10-20)
(Optional)

Cardio Done Today:

....

Workout 62

Chest **& Biceps**

1. Doorway Curl

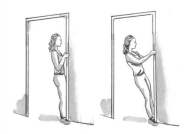

Previous Best
(Workout 57)   Reps: ....

Set 1   Reps: ....   (Goal: 10-20)

Set 2   Reps: ....   (Goal: 10-20)

Set 3   Reps: ....   (Goal: 10-20)

Set 4   Reps: ....   (Goal: 10-20)
(Optional)

2. Flexing Hammer Curl

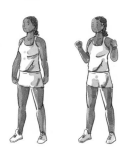

Previous Best
(Workout 57)   Reps: ....

Set 1   Reps: ....   (Goal: 10-20)

Set 2   Reps: ....   (Goal: 10-20)

Set 3   Reps: ....   (Goal: 10-20)

Set 4   Reps: ....   (Goal: 10-20)
(Optional)

3. Curl Your Leg

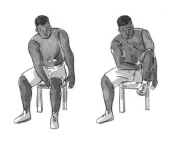

Previous Best
(Workout 57)   Reps: ....

Set 1   Reps: ....   (Goal: 10-20 Each Side)

Set 2   Reps: ....   (Goal: 10-20 Each Side)

Set 3   Reps: ....   (Goal: 10-20 Each Side)

Set 4   Reps: ....   (Goal: 10-20 Each Side)
(Optional)

4. Towel Curl

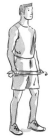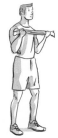

Previous Best
(Workout 57)   Reps: ....

Set 1   Reps: ....   (Goal: 10-20)

Set 2   Reps: ....   (Goal: 10-20)

Set 3   Reps: ....   (Goal: 10-20)

Set 4   Reps: ....   (Goal: 10-20)
(Optional)

Supersets Done Today (Circle):

1   2   3   4

 Today's Workout Intensity:

............../10

Shoulders & Triceps

1. Y Raises

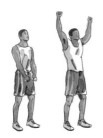

Previous Best
(Workout 58)   Reps: ....

Set 1   Reps: .... (Goal: 10-20)

Set 2   Reps: .... (Goal: 10-20)

Set 3   Reps: .... (Goal: 10-20)

Set 4   Reps: .... (Goal: 10-20)
(Optional)

2. Towel Snatch

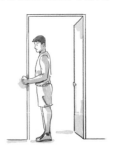

Previous Best
(Workout 58)   Reps: ....

Set 1   Reps: .... (Goal: 10-20)

Set 2   Reps: .... (Goal: 10-20)

Set 3   Reps: .... (Goal: 10-20)

Set 4   Reps: .... (Goal: 10-20)
(Optional)

3. Doorframe Hold

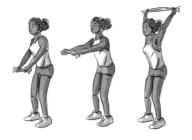

Previous Best
(Workout 58)   Reps: ....

Set 1   Reps: .... (Goal: 10-20 Each Side)

Set 2   Reps: .... (Goal: 10-20 Each Side)

Set 3   Reps: .... (Goal: 10-20 Each Side)

Set 4   Reps: .... (Goal: 10-20 Each Side)
(Optional)

4. Pike Push Up

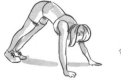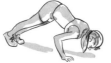

Previous Best
(Workout 58)   Reps: ....

Set 1   Reps: .... (Goal: 10-20)

Set 2   Reps: .... (Goal: 10-20)

Set 3   Reps: .... (Goal: 10-20)

Set 4   Reps: .... (Goal: 10-20)
(Optional)

    Cardio Done Today:

....

Shoulders **& Triceps**

1. Bodyweight Dips

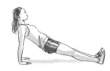
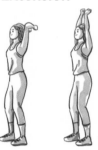

Previous Best
(Workout 58)   Reps: ....

Set 1   Reps: ....   (Goal: 10-20)

Set 2   Reps: ....   (Goal: 10-20)

Set 3   Reps: ....   (Goal: 10-20)

Set 4   Reps: ....   (Goal: 10-20)
(Optional)

2. Flexing Overhead Tricep Extension

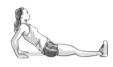

Previous Best
(Workout 58)   Reps: ....

Set 1   Reps: ....   (Goal: 10-20)

Set 2   Reps: ....   (Goal: 10-20)

Set 3   Reps: ....   (Goal: 10-20)

Set 4   Reps: ....   (Goal: 10-20)
(Optional)

3. Bodyweight Skull Crusher

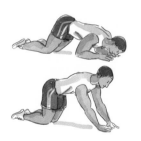

Previous Best
(Workout 58)   Reps: ....

Set 1   Reps: ....   (Goal: 10-20)

Set 2   Reps: ....   (Goal: 10-20)

Set 3   Reps: ....   (Goal: 10-20)

Set 4   Reps: ....   (Goal: 10-20)
(Optional)

4. Diamond Push Up

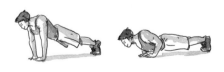

Previous Best
(Workout 58)   Reps: ....

Set 1   Reps: ....   (Goal: 10-20)

Set 2   Reps: ....   (Goal: 10-20)

Set 3   Reps: ....   (Goal: 10-20)

Set 4   Reps: ....   (Goal: 10-20)
(Optional)

Supersets Done Today (Circle):

1   2   3   4

Today's Workout Intensity:

............../10

<u>Legs</u> & Abs

1. Bodyweight Deadlift

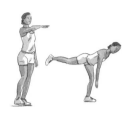

Previous Best
(Workout 59)   Reps: ....

    Set 1   Reps: ....   (Goal: 10-20 Each Side)

    Set 2   Reps: ....   (Goal: 10-20 Each Side)

    Set 3   Reps: ....   (Goal: 10-20 Each Side)

    Set 4   Reps: ....   (Goal: 10-20 Each Side)
    (Optional)

2. Glute Bridge

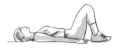
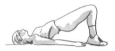

Previous Best
(Workout 59)   Reps: ....

    Set 1   Reps: ....   (Goal: 10-20)

    Set 2   Reps: ....   (Goal: 10-20)

    Set 3   Reps: ....   (Goal: 10-20)

    Set 4   Reps: ....   (Goal: 10-20)
    (Optional)

3. Curtsy Lunge

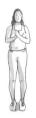
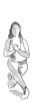

Previous Best
(Workout 59)   Reps: ....

    Set 1   Reps: ....   (Goal: 10-20 Each Side)

    Set 2   Reps: ....   (Goal: 10-20 Each Side)

    Set 3   Reps: ....   (Goal: 10-20 Each Side)

    Set 4   Reps: ....   (Goal: 10-20 Each Side)
    (Optional)

4. Tabletop + Donkey Kick

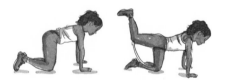

Previous Best
(Workout 59)   Reps: ....

    Set 1   Reps: ....   (Goal: 10-20 Each Side)

    Set 2   Reps: ....   (Goal: 10-20 Each Side)

    Set 3   Reps: ....   (Goal: 10-20 Each Side)

    Set 4   Reps: ....   (Goal: 10-20 Each Side)
    (Optional)

5. Calf Raise

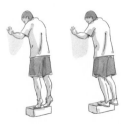

Previous Best
(Workout 59)   Reps: ....

    Set 1   Reps: ....   (Goal: 10-20)

    Set 2   Reps: ....   (Goal: 10-20)

    Set 3   Reps: ....   (Goal: 10-20)

    Set 4   Reps: ....   (Goal: 10-20)
    (Optional)

 Cardio Done Today:

....

Legs **& Abs**

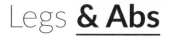

1. Spider-Man Plank Crunch

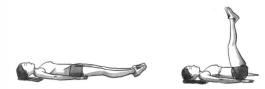

Previous Best
(Workout 61)   Reps: ....

Set 1	Reps:	(Goal: 10-20 Each Side)
Set 2	Reps:	(Goal: 10-20 Each Side)
Set 3	Reps:	(Goal: 10-20 Each Side)
Set 4 (Optional)	Reps:	(Goal: 10-20 Each Side)

2. Leg Lift

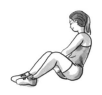

Previous Best
(Workout 61)   Reps: ....

Set 1	Reps:	(Goal: 10-20)
Set 2	Reps:	(Goal: 10-20)
Set 3	Reps:	(Goal: 10-20)
Set 4 (Optional)	Reps:	(Goal: 10-20)

3. Russian Twist

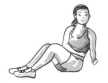

Previous Best
(Workout 44)   Reps: ....

Set 1	Reps:	(Goal: 10-20 Each Side)
Set 2	Reps:	(Goal: 10-20 Each Side)
Set 3	Reps:	(Goal: 10-20 Each Side)
Set 4 (Optional)	Reps:	(Goal: 10-20 Each Side)

4. Plank

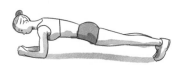

Previous Best
(Workout 61)   Reps: ....

Set 1	Time:	(Goal: 45-90 Seconds)
Set 2	Time:	(Goal: 45-90 Seconds)
Set 3	Time:	(Goal: 45-90 Seconds)
Set 4 (Optional)	Time:	(Goal: 45-90 Seconds)

Supersets Done Today (Circle):

1   2   3   4

 Today's Workout Intensity:

................/10

Full Body Workout

Exercise Guide
https://habitnest.link/WGBJ-BW65

Rest for **15-20 seconds between each exercise**, then rest for **1-2 minutes after completing** the entire circuit. Complete the full circuit **a total of 4-5 times**.

1. Run In Place

30 seconds

2. Mountain Climber

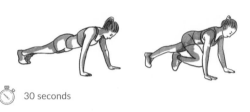

30 seconds

3. Starfish Crunch

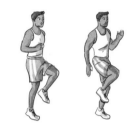

30 seconds

4. Bicycle Crunch

30 seconds

5. Alternating Lunge

30 seconds

6. Towel Snatch

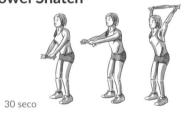

30 seco

7. Push Up

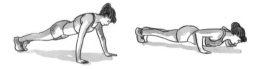

30 seconds

8. Vertical Leap

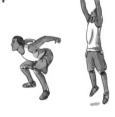

30 seconds

Circuits Completed (Circle):   196   Today's Workout Intensity:

1   2   3   4   5   ..../10

Congratulations!!!

You've made it to the end of the journal and completed an INTENSE body sculpting regimen that has no doubt increased your strength, appearance, confidence, and ability to accomplish your goals.

For you to have gotten this far means you've earned a very serious congratulations. You need to celebrate because your willpower and confidence should be soaring through the roof.

You've gained lessons about yourself not many dare to approach. You've struggled with your own mind, body and heart and gained some serious control over them. You fully understand that you have the power in you to accomplish ANY goal you put your mind to.

That's so awesome. You are a true WARRIOR.

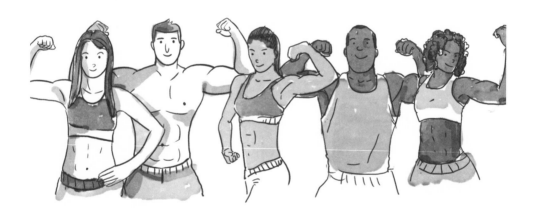

Note: We LOVE sharing stories of our users and what their lives looked like BEFORE using the journal compared to where they are NOW!

If you want to share your story with us, you can do so here: habitnest.com/bodyweighttestimonial

Check-In

How has my life changed since I started this program?

....
....
....

What changes have I seen in my attitude?

....
....
....

What physical changes have I seen?

....
....
....

How do I feel about myself in general compared to when I started this program?

....
....
....

How do I see myself continuing to build on what I've learned and gained by doing this program?

....
....
....

- Fin -

So... What Now?

Although you should feel very accomplished for getting through this entire journal... know that you built this habit to continually improve your life. Don't stop now. This is only the beginning.

One huge factor to this is tracking your progress. Once you stop tracking, it makes it exponentially easier for you to skip having a consistent workout practice (due to the lack of accountability with yourself).

Remember: **Every single day in your life where you incorporate a strong foundation of fitness will automatically be a better day of your life.**

You only stand to gain from continuing this habit.

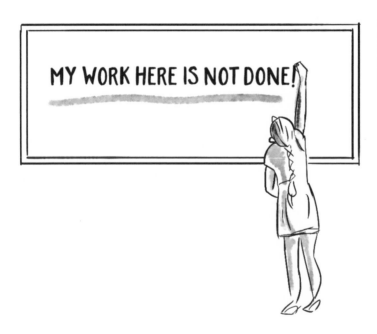
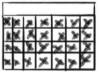

Continuing the Habit

The first question we get from users who finish the journal is 'what should I do now?' For that reason we have an array of weight-training journals in the Weightlifting Gym Buddy Journal series!

If you think it'd be useful for you to continue growing with this practice, you can find out more here: **habitnest.com/weightliftingseries**

The series includes:

- **The Weightlifting Gym Buddy Journal – Volume I**
- **The Weightlifting Gym Buddy Journal – Volume II**
- **The Weightlifting Gym Buddy Journal – Volume III**
- **The Weight Training Tracker**

Each one of these journals requires access to a gym.

The Volumes gradually increase the difficulty of each workout as time goes on, helping to promote continual muscle development and introduce further variety to your workouts.

By the time you complete all three starting journals, you will have found which exercises have been most impactful for you and your progress. The final journal, The Weight Training Tracker, becomes a blank canvas for you to design your own workouts each day and follow along from there.

If you feel it would be helpful to continue this practice and tracking your progress, these are the tools for you.

You can get yours here! **habitnest.com/ weightliftingseries**

Meet the Habit Nest Cofounders

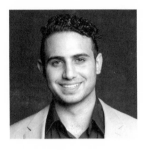

Amir Atighehchi

Amir graduated from USC's Marshall School of Business in 2013. He got his first taste of entrepreneurship during college with Mikey when they co-founded a bicycle lock company called Nutlock. It wasn't until after college when he opened his eyes to the world of personal development and healthy habits. Amir is fascinated by creative challenges and entrepreneurship.

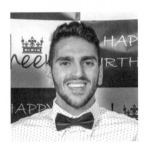

Mikey Ahdoot

Mikey transformed his life from a 200+ pound video game addict to someone who was doing 17 daily habits consistently at one point. From ice cold showers to brainstorming 10 ideas a day (shoutout to James Altucher) to celebrating life every single day, he is first hand becoming a habit routine machine that sets himself up for success daily. He is a graduate of USC's Marshall School of Business and a proud Trojan.

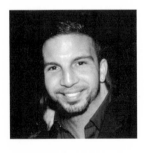

Ari Banayan

Ari graduated from the University of Southern California Gould School of Law in 2016. Through his own life experience, he understands how important it is to take care of ourselves mentally, physically and emotionally to operate at maximum capacity. He uses waking up early, reading, meditation, exercise, and a healthy diet to create a solid foundation for his everyday life.

Read all of our full stories here:
habitnest.com/aboutus

Shop Habit Nest Products

Lifestyle Products

*All of our lifestyle journals come with **daily content** (including Pro-Tips, Daily Challenges, Practical Resources, & more) to inspire you and give you bite-sized information to use along your journey. They also contain **daily questions aimed at holding you accountable** to ingraining that habit into your life.*

- ***The Morning Sidekick Journal Series***
  A set of guided morning planners that help you conquer your mornings and conquer your life. This complete 4-volume series covers 1-year of morning routines.

- ***The Evening Routine / Sleep Sidekick Journal***
  Helps you to wind down your days peacefully, prepare for each next day, and get the most rejuvenating sleep of your life.

- ***The Gratitude Sidekick Journal***
  A research-based journal that will help make an **attitude of appreciation** a core part of who you are.

- ***The Meditation Sidekick Journal***
  Built to give you all the tools you need to stay consistent with a meditation practice.

- ***The Nutrition Sidekick Journal***
  Your nutrition tracker, informational guide, and coach, all in one.

- ***The Budgeting Sidekick Journal Series***
  The most simple-yet-effective budgeting guide in the world, helping you find full clarity on your budgeting goals and to achieve financial freedom. Set spending goals, track your daily spending, and reconcile along the way. Contains 2 volumes which cover well over a year of budgeting.

Fitness Products

Our no-nonsense fitness books have fully guided fitness routines.
No thinking required; just open the books and follow along.

- **The Weightlifting Gym Buddy Journal Series**
A set of guided personal training programs aimed at helping you have the best workouts of your life. This complete 4-volume series covers 1-year of weightlifting workouts.

- **The Bodyweight / Dumbbell Home Workout Journals**
Specifically focus on HOME workout programs that require minimal-to-no equipment to complete.

- **The Badass Body Goals Journal**
An at-home-friendly fitness journal that focuses on HIIT and circuit workouts. This journal comes with a full video guide you can play and follow along.

Other Products

- **The Habit Nest Mobile Application**
The app will offer a digital representation of our journals so you can stay on your Habit Nest journey while mobile. Available on iOS & Android.

- **The Habit Nest Daily Planner**
Plan your day including your top priorities, smaller 5-minute tasks, and all your to-dos. Get optional suggestions for ways to start your mornings and end your evenings with as well.

- **George The Short-Necked Giraffe (Children's Book)**
Follow along George's journey as he learns the hard way that fully accepting himself, exactly the way he is, is the only path to living his happiest life.

Shop all products here: **habitnest.com/store**

Share the Love

If you're reading this, that means you've come pretty far from where you were a couple months ago. You should be extremely proud of yourself!

If you believe this journal has had a positive impact on your life, we invite you to consider gifting a new one to a friend.

Is there a holiday coming up? Is there a special birthday around the corner? Or do you just want to put a smile on someone's face and do something incredible for them?

Gifting this journal is the absolute best way to show any gratitude you may have for what we've written here, as well as serving as a force of good through giving back to others. And you can rest assured that you're helping improve another person's life at the same time.

We created a discount code for getting this far that can be used for any Gym Buddy Journal or Home Workout Journal reorder (make sure to use the same email address you placed the order with).

If you decide to, feel free to re-order here:
habitnest.com/weightlifting
Use code **Gains16** for **16% off!**

The Habit Nest Mobile App

When Habit Nest was initially founded, it was supposed to be in mobile app form from the start. We tried for a year as a team of three young founders with no outside funding to get a mobile app built, but we never could pull it off back then.

We switched to paper journals that worked using the same concept, which you're currently holding. Now, 5 years and hundreds of thousands of journals sold later, **we're finally in a place to chase our dream** of creating an app.

It's making us a bit emotional as things have come full circle and we're unbelievably **thankful for every single customer (like you)** who has helped us get here, shared their ups and downs with us, and really just **given us a chance** to grow our little company that sincerely cares.

We've been working extremely hard to be able to create the Habit Nest mobile app this year and **it will be live in the iOS and Android app stores in January 2021.**

The app will offer a **digital representation of our journals** so you can stay on your Habit Nest journey while mobile.

If you're interested in seeing how it can help you, feel free to see more at **habitnest.com/app**

Thank you for making this possible.

With hugs and a lot of love,
Mikey Ahdoot, Ari Banayan, & Amir Atighehchi
Cofounders of Habit Nest

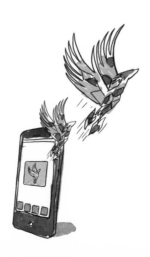

Content Index

Workout Index

Ab Workouts

Bicycle Crunch

1. Lie flat with your lower back pressed to the ground. Place your hands behind your head slightly above your neck. Lift your shoulders into a crunch position.

2. Raise yours legs so that your thighs are perpendicular to the ground and your shins parallel to the ground.

3. Simultaneously, slowly go through a cycle pedal motion kicking forward with the right leg while pulling in the knee of the left leg.

4. Bring your right elbow close to your left knee by crunching to the side. Then crunch to the opposite side as you cycle your legs and bring your left elbow closer to your right knee.

5. Alternate sides.

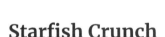

Starfish Crunch

1. Lie on your back with your arms and legs stretched out into an 'X' position.

2. In one movement, bring one arm straight up across your body while simultaneously lifting your opposing leg and lifting your head.

3. Attempt to touch one arm to your opposite ankle, or try to come as close as you can.

4. Alternate sides.

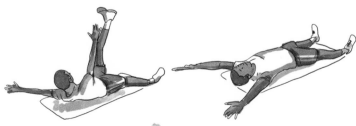

Ab Workouts

Leg Lift

1. Lie with your back flat on the floor (or on a bench) with your legs extended in front of you.

2. Place your hands to your sides with your palms facing down. To keep your hands down for support, you can place them under your glutes.

3. Keep your legs fully extended and as straight as possible (it's okay if your knees slightly bend). Hold the contraction at the top for a second.

4. Slowly lower your legs back down to the starting position.

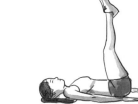

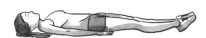

Plank

1. Place your forearms on the ground with your elbows aligned beneath your shoulders. Keep your arms parallel to your body at about shoulder-width distance. (You should be in a push up position, only on your forearms rather than your hands).

2. Ground your toes into the floor and squeeze your glutes to stabilize your body. Be careful to not to lock or hyperextend your knees.

3. Neutralize your neck and spine by looking at a spot on the floor about a foot in front of your hands. Your head should be in line with your back. Contract your abdominals to keep yourself up and prevent your booty from sticking up.

4. Keep your back flat and hold the position for as long as possible without compromising form.

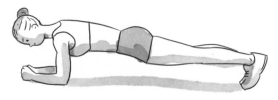

Ab Workouts

Russian Twist

1. Lie down on the floor placing your feet either under something that will not move or by having a partner hold them. Your legs should be bent at the knees.

2. Elevate your upper body so that it creates an imaginary V-shape with your thighs. Your arms should be fully extended in front of you perpendicular to your torso and with the hands clasped. This is the starting position.

3. Twist your torso to the right side until your arms are parallel with the floor while breathing out.

4. Hold the contraction for a second and move back to the starting position while breathing out.
   Now move to the opposite side performing the same techniques you applied to the right side.

5. Repeat for the recommended amount of repetitions.

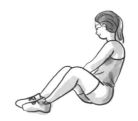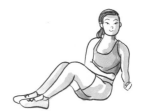

Spider-Man Plank Crunch

1. Get in plank position by placing your elbows and toes on the floor. Hold your body up off the floor in this position.

2. Bring your right knee on the outside of your body to your right elbow.

3. Straighten your right leg back to the floor.

4. Complete the same movement with your left leg and keep alternating sides.

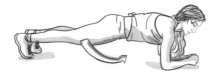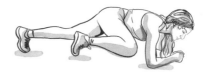

Back Workouts

Superman

1. Lie face down on the ground, toes pointed, ankles touching the ground, arms extended forward, like Superman in flight, palms down, touching the ground.

2. Pull your arms and legs off the ground by engaging your glutes, shoulders, core, and back. They should raise up 2-3 inches.

3. Ensure that your arms are also fully contracted.

4. Hold this position for 1-2 seconds.

5. Slowly lower your arms and legs back to the starting position. Repeat for prescribed number of reps.

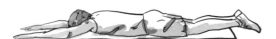
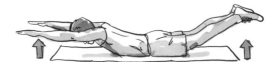

Aquaman

1. Lie face down on the ground, toes pointed, ankles touching the ground, arms extended forward, like Superman in flight, palms down, touching the ground.

2. Pull one arm and the opposite leg off the ground by engaging your glutes, shoulders, core, and back. They should raise up 2-3 inches.

3. Ensure that your arms are also fully contracted.

4. Hold this position for 1-2 seconds.

5. Slowly lower your arm and leg back to the starting position. Repeat, using the other arm and opposite leg. This is one rep.

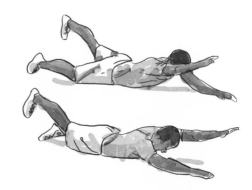

Back Workouts

Simulated Pull Up

1. Grab a towel or t-shirt, hold it in both hands, and stand in a squat position.

2. Hold the towel out in front of you with your arms extended, and pull on both sides of the t-shirt or towel as hard, as you can as if you were trying to rip it.

3. As you continue to try to rip the towel or t-shirt, slowly bring your elbows backwards as if you were trying to squeeze your shoulder blades together.

4. When your hands get as close to your chest as possible, slowly return to the starting position and repeat until the set is complete. Remember to KEEP trying to rip the towel throughout the entire exercise.

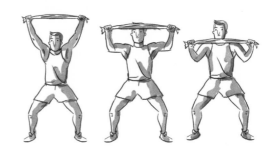

Good Morning

1. With feet hip-width apart, stand upright, knees slightly bent, and place your hands at the back of your head, elbows opened wide.

2. Engage your abdominal muscles by pulling them into your spine. Keeping your spine neutral and pressing your rear backward, bend forward at the hips and continue doing so until your back is nearly parallel to the floor.

3. Slowly return to standing, engaging your core and squeezing your glutes at the top of the movement. Continue for the prescribed number of repetitions.

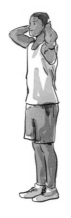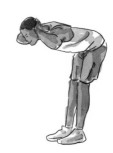

Back Workouts

Front-to-Back Towel Pull

1. Grab a towel or t-shirt, hold it in both hands, and stand in a squat position.

2. Hold the towel out in front of your chest with your arms extended, and pull on both sides of the t-shirt or towel as hard, as you can as if you were trying to rip it.

3. As you continue to try to rip the towel or t-shirt, slowly bend your elbows and bring the towel toward your chest, as if you were doing a barbell press. This is one rep.

4. Repeat as prescribed.

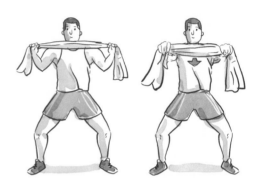

Doorway Row

1. Stand on the outside of an open doorway, facing the doorway.

2. Grip the doorjamb with each hand, palms facing outward.

3. With feet together and knees slightly bent, slowly lean your upper body back, away from the doorjamb, until your arms are straight. Your arm & back muscles should be supporting the weight of your upper body.

4. Using your lats, other supporting back muscles, and biceps pull yourself up toward the door, ensuring that your shoulder blades are pulling toward one another. This is one rep.

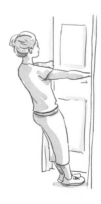
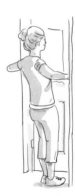

Back Workouts

Scapular Push Up

1. Position yourself as though you were going to perform a plank, hands directly beneath shoulders, arms straight, feet hip-width apart, balancing on toes.

2. Exhale. Push your shoulder blades apart as if your shoulders are moving closer to the ground. This movement will cause your upper back to rise slightly toward the ceiling.

3. Ensure that your core is engaged and arms are still straight, inhale. Bring your shoulder blades back toward each other without changing the rest of your body's position.

*Note: This can be done on the knees instead of toes.

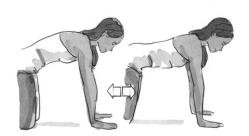

Reverse Snow Angel

1. Position yourself face-down on the floor with arms stretched out in front of you, palms facing the floor, legs closed.

2. Slowly lift your chest, arms, and legs slightly off of the ground.

3. Slowly so as to feel the tension and resistance, move your arms down toward the hips and legs outward, and then return to the original position, as though you're performing jumping jacks or a snow angel.

4. Rest limbs on the ground briefly before beginning the next rep.

*Note: If you perform this on a wood or otherwise smooth floor, you can place washcloths under your palms and toes and complete the reps without lifting your limbs off of the floor.

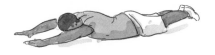

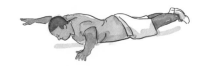

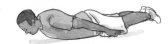

Bicep Workouts

Flexing Curl

1. Stand, with knees slightly bent.

2. Flex the muscles in your right arm, clench your fist. Slowly curly your arm upward, keeping it squeezed and under tension throughout the lift.

3. At the peak of the movement, when your hand is next to your shoulder, maintain the squeeze, and then slowly allow your arm to return.

4. Do this with the other arm.

5. Repeat!

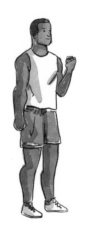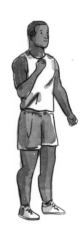

Flexing Hammer Curl

1. Stand upright with your feet shoulder-width apart. Your elbows should be tucked in close to your torso and your palms should be facing your torso.

2. Keep your upper arm stationary as you contract your biceps and curl your arms directly upward. Continue to raise your arms until your biceps are fully contracted and your wrist is at shoulder-level. Focus on only moving your forearm. Keep the muscle flexed!

3. After a brief pause, slowly begin to lower your arms back down to the starting position.

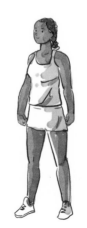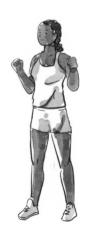

Bicep Workouts

Towel Curl

1. Grab a towel or t-shirt, hold it in both hands, palms facing upward and stand with knees slightly bent, feet hip-width apart.

2. Hold the towel out in front of you with your arms extended, and pull on both sides of the t-shirt or towel as hard, as you can as if you were trying to rip it.

3. As you continue to try to rip the towel or t-shirt, slowly curl your arms toward your body, as though you were curling a barbell.

4. When your hands reach your chest, slowly return to the starting position and repeat until the set is complete. Remember to KEEP trying to rip the towel throughout the entire exercise.

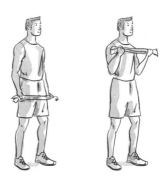

Doorway Curl

1. Stand in a doorway, facing the doorjamb, one foot in the doorway, the other on the outside of it.

2. With your hands positioned at chest-height, grip the doorjamb. Position your feet so they're close to the doorjamb and in a narrow stance.

3. Lean your body back, extending your arms. This is your starting position.

4. Engage your biceps and slowly pull your body toward the doorjamb. When you reach the doorjamb, contract your muscle. This is one rep.

*Note: For added challenge, step closer to the doorjamb or even straddle the wall with your feet.

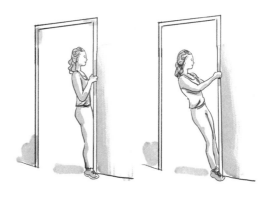

Bicep Workouts

Side-Lying Bicep Curl

1. Lie on your right side, hips and knees flexed, cushion beneath your right elbow.

2. Using your right hand, grasp your right thigh, just under the knee.

3. Let your left hand rest comfortably on your body.

4. Exhale. Raise your torso by flexing your bicep to pull.

5. Squeeze your biceps and hold this position for two seconds.

6. Inhale. Slowly lower your torso to starting position while maintaining tension.

7. This is one rep. Repeat for the opposite side.

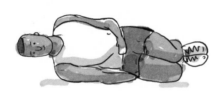
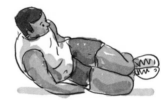

Bicep Workouts

Curl Your Leg

1. Sit in a chair with feet comfortably on the ground.

2. Take your right hand and grasp your left leg, under the knee. Your leg will serve as your resistance weight. Ensure that your leg remains "dead weight" through this exercise.

3. Engage your bicep muscles in your left hand and lift your right leg. Hold for a count of two, keeping your bicep contracted throughout the movement.

4. Return to starting position. Repeat for the opposite side.

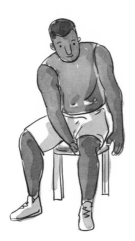 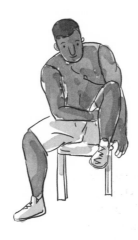

Chest Workouts

Reverse-Grip Push Up

1. Position yourself in a push-up position.

2. Rotate your wrists so that your fingertips are pointing toward your feet (depending on flexibility, you can also choose to perform this with fingertips pointing out to the sides or anywhere in between).

3. Inhale and bend your elbows and lower your chest toward the ground.

4. Push off the ground, while engaging your biceps, chest, and shoulder muscles as you slowly push off and come back to the starting position.

Note: This can be done on the knees instead of toes. It can also be done standing with hands on a wall, utilizing the same movements.

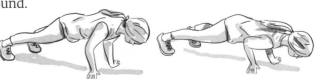

Push Up

1. Lie on the ground face down and place your hands shoulder width apart. Push your body off the ground through your hands while keeping your back as straight as possible.

2. Lower yourself back down until your chest nearly touches the ground as you inhale.

3. Exhale and press your upper body back up to the starting position while squeezing your chest, arms, and abdominal muscles.

*Note: This can be done on the knees instead of toes.

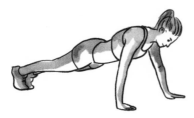
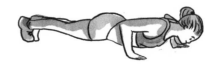

Chest Workouts

Wide-Stance Push Up

1. Begin in plank position, hands more than shoulder-width apart. For variation, you can point fingers straight ahead or turned a bit to the outside.

2. Bend your elbows slowly as you lower your body toward the floor.

3. When your chest reaches just below your elbows, pause for a count of two.

4. Contract your core muscles, press your hands into the ground, and lift your body back to start.

Note: This can be done on the knees instead of toes.

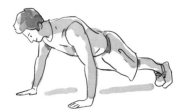 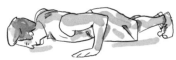

Narrow-Stance Push Up

1. Begin in plank position, hands a few inches apart from each other. The closer they are to each other, the more difficult this exercise will be.

2. Bend your elbows slowly as you lower your body toward the floor.

3. When your chest reaches just below your elbows, pause for a count of two.

4. Contract your core muscles, press your hands into the ground, and lift your body back to start.

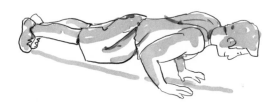

Chest Workouts

Incline Push Up

1. Stand facing a sturdy ottoman, bed, couch, bench, etc.

2. Position your hands on the edge of the furniture, slightly more than shoulder-width apart, ensuring that your elbows are not locked in place. Step your feet back until your back is straight and you are resting on the balls of your feet. This is your starting position.

3. Keeping your body straight through the entire exercise, lower yourself down toward the furniture slowly and with control until your chest touches the furniture.

4. Push your body upward, away from the furniture until you reach the original position. Do this to failure for each set. Note: This can be done on the knees instead of toes.

*Try different heights of furniture for variety and to utilize slightly different muscles each time.

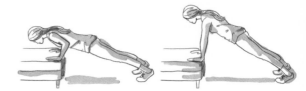

Decline Push Up

1. Begin on hands and knees, hands on the ground at shoulder-width or slightly wider (you won't want to go wider than this or your range of motion will be severely limited).

2. Lift one leg and position it atop a sturdy piece of furniture (bench, ottoman, etc.). Do this for the other leg. Ensure that your body is in a straight line before continuing. Pay attention to hips and buttocks and ensure that they aren't caving or arching. Double check hand placement and ensure that arms are extended.

3. Bend at the elbow and allow your chest to lower. You'll find yourself looking upward slightly. This is normal, just ensure that you don't try to compensate the movement with your back or buttocks.

4. Push yourself back to the starting position, being careful not to lock your elbows. This is one rep.

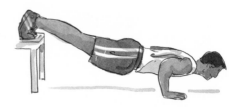

Chest Workouts

Prayers

1. Stand upright with your knees slightly bent.

2. Place your hands together in a praying position in front of your chest. Your elbows should be pointing out to your sides and your fingers pointing ahead of you while pushing tightly against each other.

3. Slowly move your hands outward away from your body so that your arms fully extend while still positioned together and pushing tightly against each other.

4. To feel this movement to its highest extent, you want to be pushing your hands together as tightly as you possible. You can try putting a weighted plate between your hands to increase the difficulty.

5. Bring your wrists back in toward your chest.

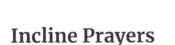

Incline Prayers

1. Stand upright with your knees slightly bent.

2. Place your hands together in a praying position in front of your chest. Your elbows should be pointing out to your sides and your fingers pointing ahead of you while pushing tightly against each other.

3. Slowly move your hands outward away from your body so that your arms fully extend, up and away from your chest, while your hands are still positioned together and pushing tightly against each other.

4. To feel this movement to its highest extent, you want to be pushing your hands together as tightly as you possible. You can try putting a weighted plate between your hands to increase the difficulty.

5. Bring your wrists back in toward your chest.

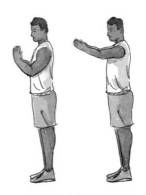

Chest Workouts

Decline Prayers

1. Stand upright with your knees slightly bent.

2. Place your hands together in a praying position in front of your chest. Your elbows should be pointing out to your sides and your fingers pointing ahead of you while pushing tightly against each other.

3. Slowly move your hands outward away from your body so that your arms fully extend, town toward your hips and away from your chest, while your hands are still positioned together and pushing tightly against each other.

4. To feel this movement to its highest extent, you want to be pushing your hands together as tightly as you possible. You can try putting a weighted plate between your hands to increase the difficulty.

5. Bring your wrists back in toward your chest.

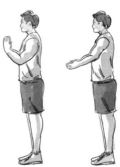

In & Out Push-Up

1. Starting out in a regular push-up position, lower the body until the elbows are bent 90° and chest is one to two inches from the ground.

2. Pressing up explosively so that the hands leave the ground. While in the air, bring the hands slightly in and back landing in close-grip push-up position, lowering down smoothly.

3. Pressing up explosively so that the hands leave the ground again and widening the grip again to go back into a regular push-up.

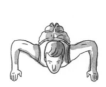

Chest Workouts

Stop-and-Release Push Up

1. Starting out in a regular push-up position, hands slightly more than shoulder-width.

2. Engage your core and lower the body all the way to the ground in a slow, controlled movement.

3. With your chest on the ground, lift your hands off the ground, squeezing shoulders together.

4. Place your palms back onto the ground and complete the push up. This is one rep.

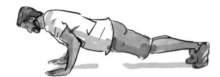 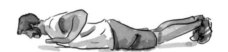

Cross-Over-Box Push Up

1. Using a sturdy box or other object, get into push up position with one hand on the box and the other hand on the floor. Your hands should be shoulder-width apart.

2. Lower yourself down as you would a typical push up, focusing on putting more of a bend in the elbow of the arm on the box than your floor-arm. The goal is to keep your chest as close to parallel with the ground as you can.

3. Push yourself back up, place the floor-hand on the box and move the box-hand onto the floor. Once both arms have performed the push up, you've completed one rep.

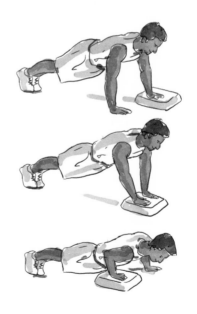

Circuit Workouts

Alternating Lunge

Caution: This movement requires a great deal of balance so if you lack balance or are suffering from an injury that affects your balance, hold on to a fixed object while completing this movement.

1. Stand with your torso upright and your hands by your sides.

2. Step forward with your right foot about 2 feet in front of you while lowering your upper body and maintaining your balance. Leave your left foot stationary behind you.

3. Squat down through your hips. Do not allow your front knee to extend beyond your toes as you lower yourself. Keep your front shin perpendicular to the ground.

4. Using mainly the heel of your foot, drive yourself back up to the starting position.

5. Alternate sides.

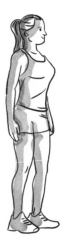

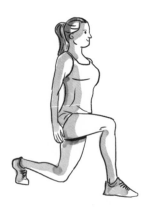

Circuit Workouts

Squat

1. Stand upright with your feet a little wider than hip-width apart and your toes turned slightly out. If you can, engage your abdominal muscles and broaden your chest by gently pulling your shoulder blades in toward each other.

2. Bend your knees slowly, pushing your glutes and hips out and down behind you as if you're sitting down on a chair. Keep your head and shoulders aligned with your knees and your knees aligned with your ankles.

3. Lower your body until your thighs are parallel to the ground. Keep your knees alined with your toes (without surpassing them) as you lower yourself as straight down as possible.

You can raise your arms up and in front of you (no higher than parallel to the ground) as you lower your body.

4. Straighten your legs to come up and squeeze your glutes as you approach the starting position.

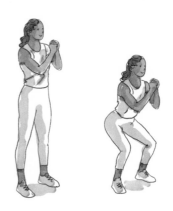

Burpee

1. Stand straight upright with both of your arms fully extended above your head.

2. Bring both hands to the ground in front of you and extend both legs straight behind you.

3. Jump or step your feet back to your hands.

4. Stand straight up and jump with your arms fully extended toward the ceiling.

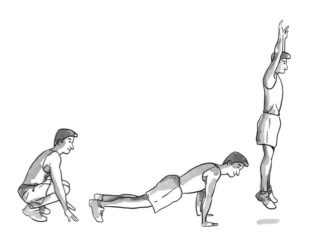

Circuit Workouts

Crunch

1. Lie on your back with your knees bent and feet resting flat on the ground hip-width apart.

2. Place your hands behind your head so that your thumbs are behind your ears.

3. Hold your elbows out to the sides and slightly tilted inward.

4. Slightly tilt your chin down, leaving a few inches of space between your chin and your chest.

5. Gently pull your abdominals inward.

6. Curl up and forward so that your head, neck, and shoulder blades lift off the ground.

7. Hold for a second at the top of the movement and then slowly lower yourself back down.

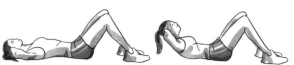

High Knee

1. Stand with your feet about shoulder-width apart.

2. Lift one leg as you drive your knee up toward your chest and raise your opposite arm. Slightly arch or round your lower back to keep your pelvis stationary and reduce strain on your back.

3. Quickly place your foot back on the ground.

4. Bring your opposite leg upward in the same motion, driving your knee to your chest, while raising your opposite arm. (This movement is essentially running in place to increase your heart rate.)

5. Alternate sides.

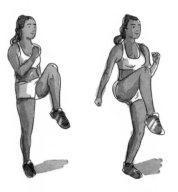

Circuit Workouts

Jump

1. Bend at the knees.

2. Jump in the air as high as you can!

3. Land softly on your feet.

4. Repeat.

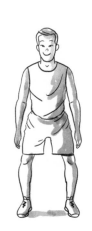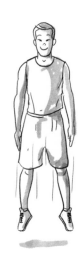

Jumping Jack

1. Stand with your feet together, knees slightly bent, and arms to your sides.

2. Jump while raising your arms and separating your legs. Land on your forefoot with your legs apart and arms overhead.

3. Jump again while lower your arms and returning your legs to midline. Land on your forefoot with your arms and legs in their original position and repeat.

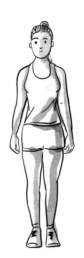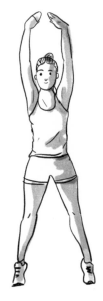

Circuit Workouts

Mountain Climber

1. Get in a push up or plank position. Keep your abdominal muscles tight and your body straight while holding yourself off the floor.

2. Pull your right knee into your chest. Make sure that your body doesn't come out of its push up or plank position. Keep your spine in a straight line and don't let your head slump. Having core body stability is very crucial for this movement.

3. Quickly place your right leg back down while simultaneously switching legs and pulling your left knee into your chest. Make sure that at the same time you push your right leg back, you pull your left knee into your chest using the same form. (This movement is essentially running in place while maintaining a straight and aligned body.)

4. Alternate sides.

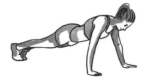 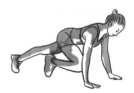

Prayers

1. Stand upright with your knees slightly bent.

2. Place your hands together in a praying position in front of your chest. Your elbows should be pointing out to your sides and your fingers pointing ahead of you while pushing tightly against each other.

3. Slowly move your hands outward away from your body so that your arms fully extend while still positioned together and pushing tightly against each other.

4. To feel this movement to its highest extent, you want to be pushing your hands together as tightly as you possible. You can try putting a 5 or 10 pound weighted plate between your hands to increase the difficulty.

5. Bring your wrists back in toward your chest.

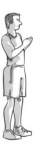 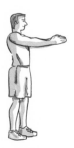

Circuit Workouts

Run In Place

1. Stand with your feet about shoulder-width apart.

2. Lift one foot off the ground by bending at the knee and repeat the motion with alternating legs.

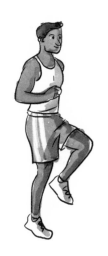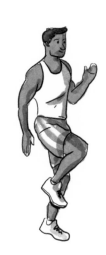

Side Plank

1. Lie down on your right side with your legs straight.

2. Prop yourself up with your right forearm so that your body forms a diagonal line.

3. Rest your left hand on your hip.

4. Brace your abdominal muscles and core.

5. Split the time between both sides of your body.

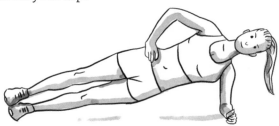

Circuit Workouts

Simulated Pull Up

1. Grab a towel or t-shirt, hold it in both hands, and stand in a squat position.

2. Hold the towel out in front of you with your arms extended, and pull on both sides of the t-shirt or towel as hard, as you can as if you were trying to rip it.

3. As you continue to try to rip the towel or t-shirt, slowly bring your elbows backwards as if you were trying to squeeze your shoulder blades together.

4. When your hands get as close to your chest as possible, slowly return to the starting position and repeat until the set is complete. Remember to KEEP trying to rip the towel throughout the entire exercise.

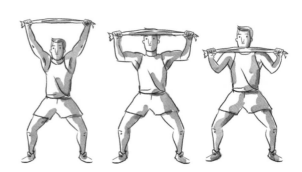

Towel Snatch

1. While holding a towel or t-shirt, get into a squat position with your feet wider than shoulder-width apart.

2. Hold the towel out in front of your body with your arms fully extended in front of you.

3. Spread your arms as if you are attempting to rip the towel in half.

4. While maintaining the squeeze of trying to rip the towel and keeping your arms straight, raise the towel up above your head and then lower it back down to the starting position.

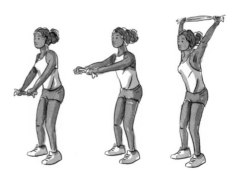

Circuit Workouts

Vertical Leap

1. Sit in a deep squat position with your weight in your heels and your booty as far back as possible.

2. Using your arms for momentum, jump up as high as you can while extending your arms to the ceiling.

3. Land in the same seated squat position that you started in.

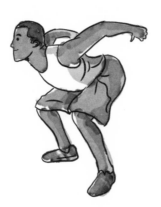
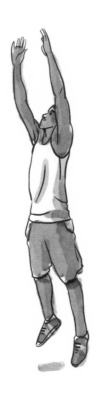

Leg Workouts

Bodyweight Deadlift

1. Stand with your feet hip-width apart. Soften your knees and shift your weight to your left leg.

2. In a controlled movement, drive your right leg behind you, hinging at the waist. Extend your left arm directly out to the side and your right arm down toward the toes on your left foot.

3. Continue tilting downward, driving your right heel back and your right hand fingertips toward your toes, until your torso is nearly parallel to the ground.

4. Lift yourself up to starting position and repeat on the opposite side. This is one rep.

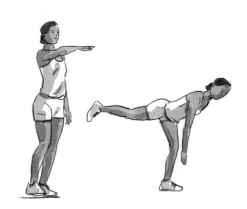

The Heisman

1. Jump or step onto your right foot and pull your left knee up towards your right shoulder as you jump.

2. Next, jump onto your left foot while bringing your right knee up towards your left shoulder.

3. Repeat the movement until the set is complete.

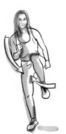 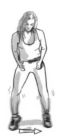 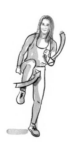 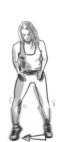

Leg Workouts

Calf Raise

1. Stand on the floor or, for more of a challenge, on a block or step, heels unsupported. (You can also do this with a weight in one hand, using the other to support your balance.)

2. Slowly lower your heels toward the floor until you feel a stretch in your calves.

3. Before your heels touch the ground, contract your calf muscles, press in to the balls of your feet, and raise yourself up until you're supporting your body with your toes, your heels raised up.

4. Repeat this, ensuring full control in all movements.

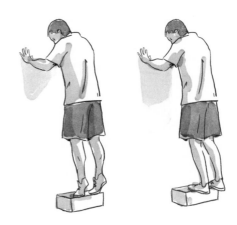

Vertical Leap

1. In a deep squat position with your weight in your heels and your booty as far back as possible, using your arms for momentum, jump up as high as you can while reaching your hands towards the ceiling.

2. Repeat this movement until the set is complete.

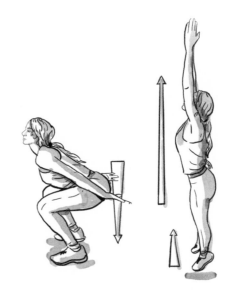

Leg Workouts

Tabletop + Donkey Kick

1. Get into a tabletop position with your hands and knees on the floor and your back comfortably straight.

2. Raise one leg and straighten it out directly behind you while raising it as high as you possibly can. Make sure to feel the contraction in your glute muscles.

3. Allow the leg to slowly return to the original position and repeat.

4. To increase the challenge of this exercise, place a weight behind your knee or utilize a resistance band on your thighs.

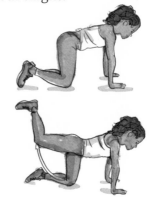

Roundhouse Kick-to-Squat

1. Get into squat position.

2. Stand straight up. As you do, shift your body to the right, raise your left foot, and kick out to the left.

3. As you're bringing your leg back to the floor, enter into the original squat position.

4. Repeat until the set is complete.

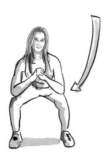
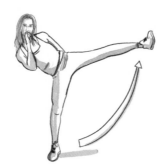
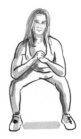

Leg Workouts

Curtsy Lunge

1. Begin by standing upright, feet hip-width apart hands either relaxed to the sides or gently clasped in front of your chest.

2. With your left foot, "draw" a semicircle until your left foot is behind your right, at a lunge-distance.

3. Drop into a lunge, as deeply as possible, without allowing your knee to touch the floor.

4. Contract your gluteal muscles and return to staring position.

5. Repeat for the opposite leg to complete one rep.

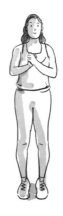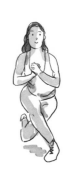

Squat

1. Stand upright with your feet a little wider than hip-width apart and your toes turned slightly out. If you can, engage your abdominal muscles and broaden your chest by gently pulling your shoulder blades in toward each other.

2. Bend your knees slowly, pushing your glutes and hips out and down behind you as if you're sitting down on a chair. Keep your head and shoulders aligned with your knees and your knees aligned with your ankles.

3. Lower your body until your thighs are parallel to the ground.

Keep your knees alined with your toes (without surpassing them) as you lower yourself as straight down as possible. You can raise your arms up and in front of you (no higher than parallel to the ground) as you lower your body.

4. Straighten your legs to come up and squeeze your glutes as you approach the starting position.

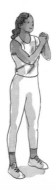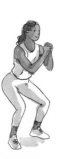

Leg Workouts

Split Squat

1. Stand with feet shoulder-width apart, hands on hips. Step one foot forward as wide as possible without losing form or balance. Ensure that your knee doesn't extend over your toes.

2. Bend both knees and lift the heel of your back foot up off of the ground, putting weight into the heel of the front foot.

3. Continue lowering your weight until your back leg shin and front leg thigh are nearly parallel to the ground.

4. Pause for a count of two. Drive the heel of the front foot into the ground and stand to return to starting position. Repeat on the opposite side for one rep.

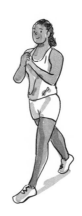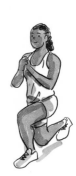

Glute Bridge

1. Position yourself with your back the ground, knees bent and feet on the floor, hip-width apart, shins perpendicular to the floor.

2. Engage your core by first flattening your back onto the ground. Imagine a string pulling your bellybutton into your spine.

3. Brace your core and drive your hips and chest upward at the same time until your torso, hips and thighs form a 45° angle to the floor.

4. Contract your glute muscles and hold for a count of 2.

5. In a controlled movement, return to starting position to begin the next rep.

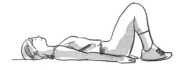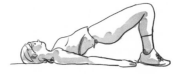

Leg Workouts

Elevated Glute Bridge

1. Position yourself with your back on the ground, heels of your feet resting on a sturdy piece of furniture (e.g. ottoman, chair, bench, etc.) and knees bent at a 90° angle.

2. Engage your core by first flattening your back onto the ground. Imagine a string pulling your bellybutton into your spine.

3. Brace your core and drive your hips and chest upward at the same time until your torso, hips, and thighs form a straight line.

4. Contract your glute muscles and hold for a count of 2.

5. In a controlled movement, return to starting position to begin the next rep.

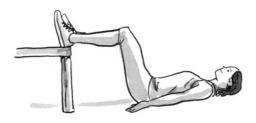

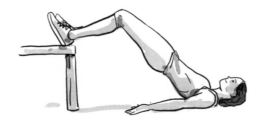

Shoulder Workouts

Towel Snatch

1. Grab a towel, t-shirt, band, or any sturdy, lightly stretchable object you can pull between your hands. Hold the ends of it and let your hands naturally drop down below your waist as if you were simply holding it.

2. Hold the object taught, as if you're attempting to rip it in half (make sure you've chosen a fabric that can withstand this).

3. As you pull it, keep you hands and arms straight and do not move your elbows. Move your hands up from your body, all the way over your head, and then bring them back towards your waist, ensuring that you are pulling the object the entire time.

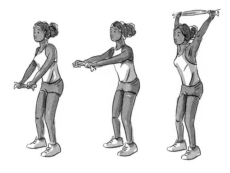

Side Plank + Twist

1. Position yourself in a side plank, left shoulder over left elbow and body in a strong, straight line.

2. Reach the fingertips of your right hand toward the ceiling.

3. Engage your core and turn your torso forward. Bring your right hand down and position it between your torso and the floor, as though you were trying to twist and reach the rest of the room behind you.

4. Slowly rotate back to starting position. Repeat on the other side to complete one rep.

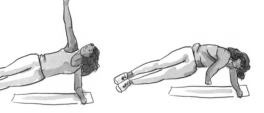

Shoulder Workouts

Reverse Push Up

1. Position yourself as though you're about to perform a traditional push up, arms extended and positioned slightly more than shoulder-width apart.

2. Bend at the knees, push your buttocks toward your ankles, pressing down on your hands, until your knees are at a 90° angle (possibly more, if you have long legs!)

3. Pause for a second, then slide your entire body forward until you are back in traditional push up position. This is one rep.

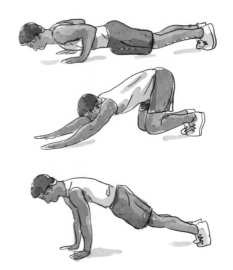

Doorframe Hold

1. Stand in a doorway, facing the doorjamb, feet hip-width apart. Bend both elbows at 90°, make a fist, and place your fists against the wall.

2. Press into the wall as if you were attempting to push through the wall and into your abdomen. Your shoulder should be engaged, but you shouldn't move your shoulder at any point during this movement.

3. Hold for a count of 5 and release. Repeat.

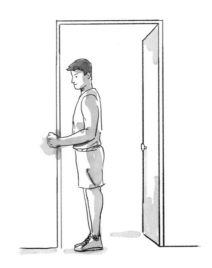

Shoulder Workouts

Arm Scissors

1. Stand upright with feet shoulder-width apart and a slight bend in the knees.

2. Stretch your arms out to your sides, parallel with the ground.

3. Engage your core and cross your arms over one another in front of your body.

4. Quickly bring them back to starting position.

5. Do the same, but alternating which arm crosses over the other. This completes one rep.

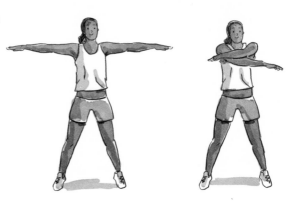

Pike Push Up

1. Position your body as though you were going to perform a plank, with your body forming a straight line from head, hips, and heels.

2. Engage your core and begin to lift your hips toward the ceiling. At the same time, walk your hands towards your feet.

3. Once your torso is nearly perpendicular to the ground, position your hands wider than your shoulders. Shift your weight to your hands and move your feet so you are on your toes.

4. Gaze toward your toes to keep your head neutral and begin to bend your elbows, lowering your head toward the floor.

5. Once you've lowered as far as you can, push yourself back up to complete one rep.

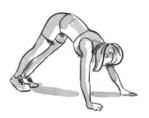 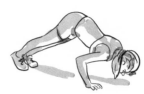

Tricep Workouts

Y Raises

1. Stand upright, feet shoulder-width apart.

2. With a slight bend in your elbows, raise your arms upward and out to the sides, making a "Y" formation until elbows are aligned with each ear. Contract shoulder muscles.

3. Slowly lower arms, maintaining control to complete one rep.

4. Remember, the point is to feel the resistance and tension. Keep your shoulder muscles flexed throughout the movement.

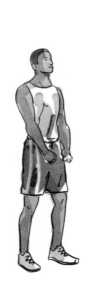
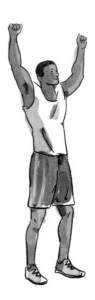

Diamond Push Up

1. Start by lying on the floor face down with your hands closer than shoulder-width apart. Hold your torso up at arm's length.

2. Lower yourself until your chest almost touches the floor.

3. Using your triceps, press your upper body back up and squeeze your chest.

*Note: This can be done on the knees instead of toes.

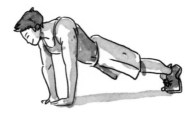
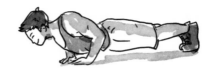

Tricep Workouts

Flexing Overhead Tricep Extension

1. Stand upright with feet positioned about shoulder-width apart.

2. Extend your arms behind your head, elbows pointing toward the sky, keeping your triceps flexed throughout the whole movement.

3. Clench your fists, as though you're trying to drive your fingers through your fist, and engage your tricep muscles. Slowly bring your forearm up until your arms are straight in the air.

4. Lower back down to starting position to complete one rep.

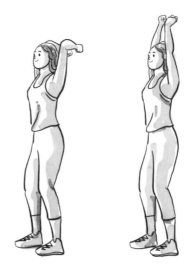

Tricep Towel Rip

1. Grab a towel, t-shirt, band, or any sturdy, lightly stretchable object you can pull between your hands.

2. Hold the ends of it at chest level, arms outstretched, but elbows slightly bent and pull the ends away from each other, as though you're attempting to rip it apart.

3. Hold for 2 counts and disengage muscles (without dropping the towel) to complete one rep.

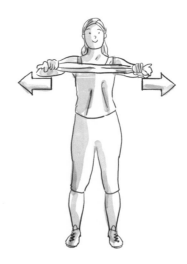

Tricep Workouts

Bodyweight Skull Crusher

1. Position yourself on your hands and knees, hands positioned slightly less than shoulder-width. Lower yourself down so that your elbows rest on the floor, positioned beneath your body, palms facing down.

2. Lean forward. Your bodyweight should be supported by your elbows.

3. Extend your elbows and push your body off of the floor. Contract your tricep muscles.

4. Flex your elbows and lower your body to the starting position to complete one rep.

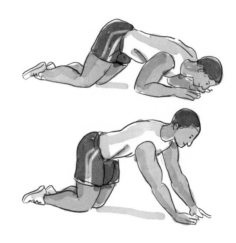

Side Tricep Extension

1. Begin on your side on the floor, bodyweight supported by your elbow, which should be positioned just beneath your shoulder. Your other arm can rest on your hip/abdomen.

2. Engage your tricep muscles, drive your forearm into the ground, and push yourself up until your hand is on the floor, supporting your bodyweight.

3. Slowly lower your arm down to starting position, with elbow on the ground. Complete prescribed number of reps on one side, before switching to the other side to round out all reps.

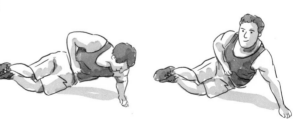

Tricep Workouts

Bodyweight Dips

1. Sit on a bench or sturdy surface (e.g. chair, box, ottoman, etc.) or simply, position yourself on the floor. Place your hands on either side of you, shoulder-width apart, fingertips curled over the edge of the furniture or palms flat on the floor, fingertips pointing toward toes.

2. Slide your buttocks off of the edge. Your legs should be straight out in front of you and your back should be close to the furniture.

3. Straighten your arms, but maintain a slight bend in your elbows.

4. Lower your body toward the ground by slowly bending your elbows.

5. Once they have formed a 90° angle, contract your tricep muscles, press the heels of your hands into the furniture and lift your body back up. This is one full rep.

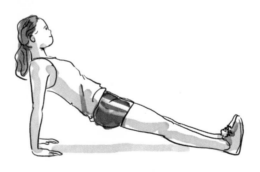

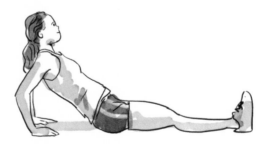